A HOSPICE CHAPLAIN'S FIELD GUIDE TO CAREGIVING

FINDING RESILIENCE ON THE FRONTLINES OF LOVE

EM HAGER

ZIP SISTERS PUBLISHING

Third Edition

ISBN-13: 978-1-882807-20-8 (Hardcover edition)

ISBN-13: 978-1-882807-04-8 (Paperback edition)

ISBN-13: 978-1-882807-02-4 (Ebook edition)

To the folks in San Francisco's Coming Home Hospice
who watched with love when I could not.

And

Albertina Xavier—1910-2017
Almost 108 years of love and wit rippling its way through the world
(Thank you for my eight—I remember.)

HOW TO USE THIS BOOK

The first eight gifts make you renewable.

If you are as stressed out as I was in caregiving, this book (any book or information) will not get into your awareness. I didn't have the receptors...my mental Wi-Fi was off.

However, if some lovely *someone buys you this book* because they are *worried* about you, try the first eight ideas only. They insure survival. They will, when practiced, get you to a more grounded place. It will give you an inner fulcrum to stand because they are about staying alive. They are also about the possibility of returning to your own center. If you go no further than this, you will benefit from increased vitality, mood, and general health.

That's enough. That's a blessing.

The first eight ideas will heal you—*enough*. This is not a guarantee, but a promise to show you how I did it while caregiving a difficult diva mother. If they work their magic on you, you will become grounded enough to make better, more loving decisions for yourself and your beloved who is infirm. Otherwise we remain too stressed and we ourselves are not only likely to fall ill, but to be ill prepared for our future life without them (...or beside them as the fates permit).

INTRODUCTION

Caregiving Could Kill You...

And it could be the best thing you have ever done, which it was for me. It will be remembered with satisfaction for the rest of my (hopefully) long and healthy life. Whichever it is, twenty-four/seven caregiving is not business as usual. It muddles everything. Its life stressors are off the charts. When I was caregiving my mother, her dementia mixed it up even more.

Yet, even if caregiving is *only* for a month, or two—a year or twelve, even if there is no dementia, this showing up in the trenches of love changes you. It can push your buttons to the extent that you may think you, yourself, are demented. It is an impossible task, which we do however we can but it is dangerous work. Statistically, we are more likely to fall sick ourselves (which I did)...and in some cases more likely to die from the delayed stress of post death caregiving (which, happily, I did not).

As we face complicated decisions and the burden of managing, we ourselves become vulnerable. It is DIY, learn as you go, a little more each day, because we must—but caregiving is *dodgy* work. We tend to allow the life and death necessities of our loved ones to take priority. We must—and yet we must not. How will we walk with them to the end (of love, life or illness) unless we do? Sound impossible? Yet, millions of us do it *every* day.

Or Caregiving Might Save You...

This book may save you by avoiding some serious mistakes—mistakes, which could damage you. However, at minimum, it will give you a reasonably good shot to be in the healthy and satisfied caregiver category. These thirty-one notions are *my rules* and gifts to you. They *generate* solutions from your core; solutions, which fit who you are and what is appropriate for your family and situation. They are inside-out principles, not those imposed upon you with completed solutions. (But, to be fair, some of the more tactical caregiving *how-to* books are *pretty* good. (Our website has a list of some of the best.)

This book is an offering of thirty-one gifts that helped me recover from being a caregiver.

I also use them at bedside *every day* as a hospice chaplain. It is my hope that they are spoken in ways that make sense to you in a spiritual but practical framework. As an Interfaith hospice chaplain, this is my solid ground—*to not know.* I support people of any faith, or no faith and all the rivers that run between those two extremes at bedside and in bereavement. It is not my job to take sides but to have confidence that there are *no* sides. However, it is *not important* for you to believe as I do. As AA friends say, the rules work 'when you work them'. However, as it did me, they may also *seep* into you like storm water becomes groundwater and simply *amend* you.

The Distillation: Inner Generative Guides to Find Your Way Home

When you take care of a loved one, the rules *change*. These thirty-one offerings are the distillation of my mother's and my experience here in the trenches of love...because what we went through *counts* for something and your experiences do, too.

All these ideas are evergreen, resilient, and self-generative (perhaps like a firefly is self-generating with its own light). It is my hope that they guide you, as they have me, in ways that access more love and balance.

Grief (and change) is not an enemy—though I feared it for years.

It can do the heavy lifting of renewal, if we let it. Be assured, the drip, drip, drip of incremental loss of a loved one through a long illness, or dementia *is* grief—*anticipatory* grief is very common in caregiving. It, and its more intense and disturbing cousin, death grief, can leverage your inner resources (and these thirty-one notions)—to do the essential work in letting go of what's not working and, possibly, renewing your life.

I like Thich Nhat Hanh's succinct accuracy in describing this spiritual paradox. His title says it all: *No Mud, No Lotus*. In other words, the blooming of the lotus is directly related to the opportunities of the muck in which it grows—the *nutrients* in that compost. They are *dependent* on each other. Hint: you are *both* the lotus, the hot mucky mess (i.e. that enzymatic poetic alchemy of the Earth). I call it *quantum compost*.

Am I nuts to say that grief can *help* us?

Nope, I am only wise in the dirty ways of *my* trenches, (which may look a lot like yours…). I think of it as composting that shit (hitting the fan…), the dead elephant (in the room) and the miscellaneous shoulds (which are liberally offered by the well-meaning, but frequently clueless).

Grief is medicine...and torture:

- Grief clarifies what is important *to you* like nothing else…
- Grief removes pretense and fosters (slapping us up side the head with) authenticity
- Grief clears space from false ideas and notions *that are no longer working* but ones for which we have yet to let go.

The Thirty-one Gifts are My Rules...

If I could have time-traveled back, to have had these rules as a guide, I would have had more fun, done better caregiving (of myself and my mother), and been less stressed-out. I also believe I would have been quicker to recover from my losses because *I grew more resilient as I cared for her*—not less.

I tried to care for Betty with eyes and heart open to a higher purpose but, truth be told, I barely kept from misplacing her in some foreign city. I did not care for my mother perfectly, but I resolved each day to do it better. I am not saying it could have been a dance (that would be demented…), but it doesn't have to be a death dirge.

When my mother, Betty, passed, I wrote until I was empty, then groped my way to a new life. As a hospice chaplain, where I find myself, I am honored each day by the bedside stories of bravery on the frontlines of love. Life is messy. Any caregiver knows that there are trenches here that are so deep they can threaten our own lives. These same experiences may also nourish us. As a former landscape architect, I have come to see it as *the garden of change*. The circle of care—love, caregiving, loss, grief, bereavement, and renewal—is best seen, I believe, as *seasons* where the light promises to come round again—*and it does.*

These gifts will help you *spring* back—daily.

Some ideas might be new to you, or some simply reminders of what you *already* know to be true. Adding more joy and love *into* the way we give care changes our world and, especially, your beloved's remaining and *precious* life. The qualities that I brought to the life and death decisions of caregiving impacted my life, even after my mother's passing.

We have earned this wisdom but if we don't add it to the next moment and practice, we are *all* Bill Murray in *Groundhog Day,* repeating errors in habitually comic and tragic scenes, while we loop or learn how to love (Andie McDowell) and get out of our own way. We re-live the moments of our lives daily over and over, until we germinate or die. This book is a field guide to weeding and planting a new life because this is your season, too, which is something we tend to forget as loyal caregivers of our beloveds.

You are not alone...and (*probably*) not going crazy.

If you are one of the 44 million unpaid caregivers on duty in the U.S.A. right now, you are already on your journey. Many millions of us are dual-processing our day jobs and watching over our beloveds who are struggling with illnesses. The notions offered here will help you navigate this best *and hardest* trip any human being may ever walk with another—to the end of time. They are about caregiving and giving care as a renewing pair and that changes the planet.

The field guide is a short book and, later, a longer story as a memoir...

It took me eleven years of caregiving, and another six years of grief to parse these experiences, to get to a place of renewal. I have condensed these seventeen years into a *short* book because who has that kind of time? I need these rules for balance (separate of our memoir: *girlQuantum,* which will come later) to *remember* a better life for myself—the one I came here to do—moment to moment.

That is the kind of time we have—moment-to-moment.

Caregiving holds its own kind of hope and grief in a dynamic balance. Its anticipatory grief pulls us into a land *between* where we must start telling (and re-telling) our story to ground us and make our changing experiences feel *real*. We are storytellers. We need stories to live. When someone dies, a story ends. Loss compels us to speak so we can make sense of our new world. It is what the bereaved must do to move through to a less dismal place than the hard winter of grief.

Your caregiving life might be outwardly confined by honor and responsibility, but with these rules, you are free in the places that matter. Your inner landscapes will be well-made, colorfully planted and ready for spring as the seasons of life offer us.

My goal for this field guide is to accompany you but it is *your journey.* We must learn to ignore those who discount our experiences and say, they have been there. (...They have not been *you, or there.*) Caregiving is a mythic underworld, which is linked to our intimate inner world where it's good to have a sympathetic guide with you—me. The 'evidence of things not seen' is not illusion, but very, very real—here in the trenches of love and loss. You are not alone, but accompanied by a crowd of witnesses--or perhaps just Betty and me (but it is *enough*).

Best blessings on your journey,

Rev. EM Hager
http://www.EMHager.com

PREFACE

THE MOST IMPORTANT QUESTION

My mother's and my story was also a prizefight. Our lifelong argument erupted as many things, but at its core, there was only one—a worldview: Betty's vs. mine. It was intimate and public: confused and loud. It was a multi-year, many-round championship boxing match, which we had from Tulsa to San Francisco, over the answer to this question:

> "The most important question a person can ask is, "Is the Universe a friendly place?"
>
> — ALBERT EINSTEIN

I say yes. These rules help me remember that friendly providence in the garden of change.

I

THE FRONTLINES

Gift 1. Wait Here

Gift 2. Stay Full

Gift 3. Etak Compass

Gift 4. Diva Breathe

Gift 5. Gratitude of Redwoods

Gift 6. Play Daily

Gift 7. Be Willing

Gift 8. Stop. Rest

1

WAIT HERE

STOP STRUGGLING. WAIT HERE FOR THE GOODNESS TO CATCH UP.

The cold ceramic floor was sucking out her warmth as we waited for the San Francisco EMTs. I touched Betty to reassure her—or me; she was icy. Her head gash would need stitches and the doctors would later find a cracked vertebra. None of it stopped her from joking about how cute the paramedics were when they did arrive.

Five Years into Caregiving with Six to Go...

"I think he's the cutest. Doesn't he look like Glen?" Or it could be H.R. or Keith or anyone on the list of my exes. It was a familiar dance. Betty was entertaining again; she was holding court. I was her captive entourage and the firefighter-paramedics were the attentive audience. She was doing a pretty good job of holding on to some dignity as well as holding off the next phase. She and I were on the same ship sailing in denial: she was not yet my child and I was not yet her parent.

Humor was even more unexpected in the emergency room.

Her healthcare workers were perplexed, then charmed by it (especially, if they saw me modeling laughter). Or they might miss the joke entirely and report me to the authorities. "My daughter beats me." Betty had said this in response to the ER staff's private questions about the source of her many bruises from nocturnal falls. When I asked her the same thing about the new bruise du jour, she'd say, "How would I know?" It was as if I had asked about a dent in the bumper of some rental car parked on the street. Maybe she was in shock or perhaps it was her natural wit, but she thought this account was *very* funny.

THE SUBSEQUENT ELDER ABUSE REPORT ON ME ESCALATED TO POLICE involvement by the time I heard about it. The hospital social worker had already vouched for me. It took a personal intervention on my behalf from our long-time internist to finally get me off the arrest list. My mother's humor was a moment of the 'old' Betty who raised me. Gratefully, her too-sharp edges that tenderized my underbelly as an adolescent were gone. Her wit lasted until the ending days.

WHAT COULD I DO? A LOT OF IT WAS FUNNY IF NOT POINTED at you.

IN CAREGIVING, EXHAUSTION SLOWED ME DOWN. I BECAME CURIOUS enough to wonder how I was going to survive this. I made a decision to claim back some of my life—the self-sustaining part of it but I never caught up with that longing, not really. I could see glimpses of a more renewable life ahead—just out of focus.

At that point, I could not imagine that Wait *Here* might be my next best move.

Wait Here

Sometimes all you can do is take off your cape and wait for it to change...My misstep, when caregiving, was *how* I waited. I pined for a different future like a kid thinks about holiday gifts in October...focused on what was lacking. Waiting like it is already Christmas morning improves outcomes. All the presents are right here and ready for me to notice and unwrap them. My questions are about how I am going to play with them rather than, do I have enough?

As fear became my compass, I could not see a path to better options.

When my world was crashing in, husband gone, brother dead, my mother in another serial EMT crisis, it *looked* like I was competently dealing as an adult, but the truth was more like ducking for (nuclear) cover under my desk. Moving forward blindly, I stumbled into the black hole of caregiving, which sucks everything nearby into its life-and-death necessities. Its gravity trumped it all—or it did for me. I lived in the future, believing it would be better...*then*. I would make a coming-from-behind-victory as a software mogul to be financially secure, find a better man who would really *see* me, find replacement family to belong to, etc. In the effort of the middle days, I looked forward to the ending days, as some vague afterlife—after Betty.

EVEN IF WE MUST WAIT, IT IS BETTER TO WAIT *HERE* AND NOW... awake to the resources within reach.

I AM REMEMBERING THOSE MOMENTS WHEN I GOT A PRESENT-TENSE view of things. Somewhere in the anguished muck of Betty's dying, we told the truth. These were moments when the past and future bracketed me. Driven by overload, or wisdom to *now* and to *here,* I found myself—*and options.* Those, unfortunately, rare moments were hyper-real and a true compass to growing a new life. I needed to wait like a cat hunts...or a seed waits out winter... or a Buddha with equanimity, or in a more Judeo-Christian framing, it is about waiting on the Lord.

> But they who wait for the Lord shall renew their strength; they shall mount up with wings like eagles; they shall run and not be weary; they shall walk and not faint.
>
> — ISAIAH 40:31, ESV

In tango, it is all about being present to the next step.

The leader moves, the follower shadows and makes a responsive step. It is a collaboration. It is attentive waiting. The follower then pauses with complete attention for the next indication from her leader. Sometimes in tango these pauses in the motion are the most delicious part of the dance. The extended freeze frame holds the tension in the stillness and calls to the next step. Residing in the present tense is like this: "Wait, *Here*."

> You do not need to leave your room. Remain sitting at your table and listen. Do not even listen, simply wait. Do not even wait, be quiet still and solitary. The world will freely offer itself to you to be

> unmasked, it has no choice, And it will roll in ecstasy at your feet.
>
> — FRANZ KAFKA, THE ZURAU APHORISMS

Wait *Here* might be your best move—an important internal shift into stillness.

Living in the future stopped me from seeing what was right in front of me—real choices, not just more-of-the-same anxious looping. *Wait Here.*

Don't just do something. Sit there.

STOP STRUGGLING. HAVE A QUANTUM OF FAITH, *WAIT HERE* FOR THE goodness to catch up.

2

STAY FULL

RUNNING ON EMPTY? STAY FULL TO DO WHAT IS YOURS TO DO TODAY...THAT'S ENOUGH.

I was not raised to wait around for someone else *to do* things for me. I was assured they wouldn't. My mother, Betty, was an action hero in her prime—always in motion and seeking more or better. In terms of husbands, more was better. She had five (but responsibly, not all at one time).

Eating Out Without Me

"I always made more money than any of them." As a CPA, Betty relentlessly kept score, but it was also about companionship. Husbands were a lifeline and referred power (that's why she liked attorneys). They were apparently easier to find than real opportunities in the accounting profession during the post-war decades. To Betty's restive credit, she embodied consideration and civility in all the divorces and endings—at least, the four for which I was present. It was a good lesson. Betty stayed friends with her exes until their deaths; she unhappily outlived them all.

Five years into my caregiving with six more to go, my mother began leveraging her dementia to continue to see those husbands. All of them were dead in my time—but not in hers. In her time traveling, she could still have dinner with them—all of them.

"John W. came by yesterday," she told me one day when I visited her in assisted living. "We went to lunch."

As usual, I played along. It seemed irrelevant to a fine moment, to share that he had been dead for sixteen years. "Oh. Where did you go?" I asked, hoping for a clue as to *when* she was remembering. Usually it was a favorite hangout. It gave me her geopositional and temporal coordinates. On occasion, I might momentarily join her there, adding bits from my own recollection of the place. "Did you have that amazing marinated wild-caught salmon?"

Or sometimes, as her illness progressed in hospice, she would be unreachable. "You don't know the restaurant." On these occasions, she explained in a tone that was one part apologetic, the other part sadness. "It's a new place, you haven't been to it yet." She was beginning to leave me behind. Our time of sharing was ending; uncertainty was expanding. Death was nearing.

In hospice, I kidded her about the husbands that she could not clearly remember. "You never got it right. You married them as trophy husbands but they thought it was the other way around."

She laughed. I did too. It felt so satisfying to be with her there with the hospice staff as witness to the joy of letting the nattering "not enoughs" go. All that mattered was our deep-hearted, grateful little chuckle together. Oddly, in letting our 'not enoughs' go, I could *fill* up. In that moment, I felt no fear. I was full.

Stay Full

When I am empty, even small stuff is an obstacle.

Like whitewater rafting, with enough water, the raft will find its way *around* the rocks, but when the river is low with 'boney water' even a small boulder will block you.

In this caregiving venture, don't make the rookie (entrepreneurial) mistake of paying yourself last and allowing your tank to run dry. (I, myself, being an unfortunate example of this…in several businesses.) It is *dodgy* management.

This middle-ground of caring is a fulcrum where you can leverage worlds.

Caring for yourself equally with the other is not an original thought, but an ancient and golden-rule balance. We make it original, each time we practice. Love your beloved as yourself. (It works for your neighbor, too.)

As a caregiver, staying full is essential, but really, when is it not?

I must stay able: loved up, prayed up, rested up, and supported in *whatever* way I can let in. That's the trick: what can you easily let in that nourishes you? Perhaps it's poetry, music, gardening, walking yourself (or the dog), playing the piano (or with the kids). A cup of tea? A good book? A bodice buster? What makes me happy? What fills me? I keep a list in my wallet and feel improved just by thinking about it, because caregiving cannot be about doing *more to fix* our loved ones. If it is, we are lost. I can never *do* enough to stop death.

YOUR SWEET PEOPLE MAY OR MAY NOT DIE TODAY—BUT IF YOU STAY full, they'll see that you will be okay. It will let them move on in peace, and that is a gift to everyone in attendance.

STAY FULL TO DO WHAT IS *YOURS* TO DO TODAY...THAT'S ENOUGH. That's a good day.

3

ETAK COMPASS

OUR LONGINGS AND DISCONTENTS ARE INNER GUIDANCE.

When I was a child, my mother seemed to always *Stay Full* and navigate obstacles *optimistically*. As an adult, I saw that she stumbled—like everyone else.

WE CANNOT ALWAYS BE CHEERFUL COHORTS AND HONOR THE ROAD —the road that no one wants to be on but everyone wants to be done with. Our journey is downhill and inward to our own shadow lands. If we are willing, and lucky, we will be accompanied by a Virgil who has been there—a fellow *'thestral' seer*. J.K. Rowling has an animal in her *Harry Potter* series, which transports students from the train (of the mundane world) to the threshold of another world, where they might learn about their magical gifts. To those innocent of death, the transport method is invisible. Only after a dear one's death, can the beast be seen.

HOW DO I *KNOW* WHAT IS THE NEXT RIGHT MOVE? IN CAREGIVING with its anticipatory grief, the world seems like a warring armada. I am navigating without my familiar landmarks—at times without *any* landmarks. The notion of navigating *with* 'what is'—that *the unseen* could be a *friendly* force—to get where I want to go was beyond my present horizon.

The ancient Micronesians know better. In canoes using only their own senses, they move in and between *oceans*. (Having little or no sense of cardinal directions myself, this is a particularly terrifying thought.)

Etak Compass

Etak is the oral tradition of Micronesian navigation, which uses no instruments or technical manuals.

It is the opposite of my umbilical GPS devices. Outrigger canoes, paddled by Palu masters, travel a mapless ocean with etak guidance. Sure, they use knowledge of stars, swells, seasons, currents and creatures of the sea and air like other navigators, but the focus and force for a Palu master is that his canoe is *stationary* —the islands move on the sea *around him*. He is the heart of it all, the core, and is as sure of this, as we Westerners are that the *canoe* is moving.

Delusional? Self-centered? The ultimate in narcissism? It has been working for their extended voyages for millennia—holding to their own center.

Caregivers know the stressors of navigating without landmarks, day after day. In the desire to be known, or loyal, or to do the right thing, I lost my bearings for such an interval that

I misplaced my center and *my world became untethered.* I was *other*-centered. A focus on self-care would have helped but it seemed, at the time, so…selfish. (Oh my, what big boundaries you have...) However, caregiving is not a sprint, and self-care is essential for the long distance journey of caregiving. Who hasn't heard this from the mouths of well-meaning observers? But how?

Our Longings and Our Discontents: Inner Guidance

Our longing and our discontents are our constantly updating how-to maps. Their voices are directly from our hearts, waiting for us to *listen*. Even if you wall them off for a lifetime, they will continue to wait for you (all the time whispering…) until you exhaust all other possibilities for authentic navigation. (Quick, somebody, anybody, tell me what to do and where to do it.) They are gold when we can start listening. Until then we are brave explorers in other people's stories but tend to lose our own God-given narratives.

We cease to *be* the hinge, but *become unhinged* or the ultimate in co-dependence—making others our center and sole focus.

For the prolonged caregiving voyage, it's a common dilemma —to misplace our center. I knew better than to make *Betty* my nucleus…but it is so easy to become disoriented in the self-sacrifice of *another* life-and-death drama. If you have your core compass anchored in someone, who is now dizzily free-floating in illness and shifting from earth to cosmos, getting lost increases to otherworldly dimensions to become a fun house (funny-farm) ride. As a hospice chaplain, I must say that this is not a *bad thing*—

to not be of this world—but it's not yet *your thing*. It is not yet your time. It's *their* journey.

> "Perfection of means and confusion of goals seems to characterize our age."
>
> — ALBERT EINSTEIN

OUR CAREGIVING GOAL IS TO PROVIDE WHAT COMFORT WE ARE ABLE and watch over them. Modern medicine has changed the face of death. Atul Gawande characterizes today's aging as 'the fade to fragility". It is no longer a cliff. Caregiving is confronted with incremental but profound choices. In this, I must remember how to *equally value* what is happening under my own skin. I must hold to the rudder of my own heart-center to stay oriented on this side of the veil, or we will *all* be lost in a vast ocean.

WHAT WOULD HAPPEN IF I WERE AS INTENT AS A PALU MASTER?

It had been a long time since I asked myself what I wanted. What if my center was my compass?

> "Small is the number of them that see with their own eyes and feel with their own hearts."
>
> — ALBERT EINSTEIN, THE WORLD AS I SEE IT

> "Let me listen to me and not to them."
>
> — GERTRUDE STEIN

I CAN TRUST IN SUCH A COMPASS—THE ETAK COMPASS.

I want to find that midpoint in myself that interconnects 'what is' to my mind, heart, and gut in such a way that I am rooted to the center of the Earth. It will steady me, when all else fails and my beloved others die (or leave).

EVEN THEN, I NAVIGATE TO *BETTER*—ONE SMALL, SWEET ISLAND AT a time.

4

DIVA BREATHE

GENEROUS PEOPLE BREATHE DEEP BUT REAL DIVAS LET IT GO. THINK PAVAROTTI.

In caregiving, even a small spark in the dark is a great mercy. Being full or running on empty is in my control (which so little else that matters is). There is always something within me to tap this sap. The unexpected frequently happens. It shifts my day and (miraculously) it twinkles back at me. This benign wink from the Universe reminds me that life is full of commas: pause, Wait *Here,* and keep breathing.

My mother was complicated and she was my hero. I would like you to know her. Through her grit and integrity, she made a good life. It was also a better world for me because of some of the things my mother didn't do. She didn't 'let the bastards get you down.' I can still hear her saying this. It was her standard pep talk. It helped. So did our camaraderie over a Hendrick's martini in a dark and upscale restaurant after a long day.

On most days, a good life was remedy enough, that and an

exceptional exhale. It sounded to most like an exasperated sigh, but I came to understand it differently. I came to remember it better.

ANY CHANGE IS CHALLENGING—ESPECIALLY ONES NOT OF YOUR OWN making—like illness.

EVEN THOSE YOU CHOOSE, CAN BE FRUSTRATING OR DANGEROUS. Unless you have lived "an interesting life" (the fortune cookie curse) as Betty did, you might not have experienced drowning in the cultural air that is supposed to support you. We "fish" (who try something new with our lives...) are more likely to glimpse the water in which we all swim—by being thrown out of the pond. If you have, you will forever see your world, differently. Trying to breathe differently—like in *air,* for example, is even more hazardous and complicated.

THE BEST FISH DON'T EVOLVE; THEY ARE AT THE TOP OF THEIR watery game; they breathe water just fine. It's those edgy fishies, having lungs or legs, who give their all for change: they innovate.

BETTY TRIED SOMETHING NEW AND LIVED A FULL LIFE. WE MET THE opposition together. I walked with her as far as I could, but she's gone now. It is my turn—to breathe fully and deeply. Betty had a good time *and* left the world just a little bit better for her daughter, son, granddaughters, grandson, and others. She took care of herself and her responsibilities.

IT WAS LIKE BREATHING FOR HER—DIVA BREATHING.

Diva Breathe

ONE OF THE FIRST RULES OF CARING FOR YOURSELF *AND OTHERS* IS an extreme exhale.

It allows for a glamorous and sensational inhale: expiration… inspiration. Let go of what is done. Be generous with your exhale.

YOU ARE FEEDING FORESTS.

I DON'T BREATHE WELL. IT'S UNCONSCIOUS.

I shallow breathe or hold my breath—never really letting things go. I only take the minimum I need because I have been *so afraid* for so long that my house of cards would collapse.

OXYGEN IS FOOD. INEFFECTIVE BREATHING IS LIKE STARVING AT your own banquet.

Breathing in is *nourishment*. Why hoard my exhale? Some wellness experts believe it is the cause of most illness. The respiratory system can eliminate 70% of our metabolic waste. Our remaining human elimination systems are defecation at only 3%, urination at 8%, and perspiration 19%. [1]

DO YOU WANT TO RUN A CLEAN SHIP OR TO LIVE IN A DIRTY HOUSE? Give a generous exhale.

Let go of what has expired and is no longer working. A structural sigh surrenders control (which we don't have) and steps you into the moment (which we do).

OXYGEN IS ENERGY. IT'S FREE AND OUR FIRST AND LAST TASTE OF this world.

Breathe in fully and we will have more than *enough* to live well, to love well, and to create—even when it's not well. It's circulation. I take it in, receiving more, and have more to give. It's physics—not even metaphysics (but that too).

NOW THAT MY MOTHER IS DEAD AND OUR ELEVEN-YEAR CARETAKING house-of-cards has collapsed, I am seeing things differently. I am breathing for me but also for the "us" of that bond, perhaps only until I figure out what is dead and what wants to live in this "good-daughter-in-mourning" that I have become. If you're still breathing, this is your season, too. Breathe it in. Breath is your first music. Listen.

GENEROUS PEOPLE BREATHE DEEP BUT REAL DIVAS LET IT GO. THINK Pavarotti.

5

GRATITUDE OF REDWOODS

ALLOW GRATITUDE TO TURN WHAT YOU HAVE INTO ENOUGH.

My mother seemed to always be out of breath and in a hurry. My diva taught me to practice brinksmanship—not meditation. She was more about self-preservation than self-compassion.

The Most Important Question To Ask When You Feel Down

Like fire, gratitude is a tool. It improves your brain chemistry, which you need to stay fit for caregiving. You know what the anti-depressant Wellbutrin does? Boosts the neurotransmitter dopamine. So does gratitude. Know what Prozac does? Boosts the neurotransmitter serotonin. So does gratitude[2]. Gratitude fights anxiety and fear.

Just asking the question, 'What am I grateful for?' does it.[2] Even on the day caregiving punches you in the belly and it feels like there's *nothing for which* to be grateful. No worries. Doesn't matter. You don't have to *find* anything. It's the *search* that counts. It's about remembering to look in the first place.

The communities of redwoods agree. Gratitude is a superpower.

Gratitude of Redwoods

What is *enough* to a redwood tree? Redwoods are giants and appear to be independent—doing it all on their own. Their true strength is dirtier and deeper. Their comparatively shallow root system extends outward *to others,* forming a network of redwoods that *share resources.* Since the Jurassic era, they have been weathering fire, drought, floods, and storms as an interconnected community. How is it possible they share widely, and yet are fed *more...and better*?

In the mud of caregiving, below ground forest ecology is relevant.

New studies show the interconnections of organisms living in the soil help trees acquire nutrients and water. The exchange of carbon and nitrogen goes back and forth between individual trees —even, in some cases, trees *of different species.*[3]

They may have less to show for it above ground, but the root systems of pre-plow prairies were even more robust. Their roots were so connected that they could be seen as *one plant* across thousands of native grassland miles. These interconnected underground systems were not about appearance, but resilience and regeneration.

These are fungal phone networks of underground communication—with their ancestors and their progeny. They are wildly connected in mystery and miracle. So are we.

Gratitude is a superpower for wherever (and when-ever) you are.

You decide whether the glass is half-empty or half-full (but drink it with close friends). Laugh until you *Cackle.*

Allow gratitude to turn what you have into *enough.*

6

PLAY DAILY

PLAYING RIGHT WHERE I AM IS THE LONG GAME—ESPECIALLY IN THE LEFTOVER MOMENTS.

My mother was smart enough to count her blessings, but she was always eager for more and better. To her credit, she believed in integral play, where she seriously applied herself.

LIKE MOST CAREGIVERS, MY MOTHER WAS ACTUALLY QUITE ISOLATED in her heyday. The professional women my mother met were rare and seen as competition. Ladies didn't mentor each other in her generation but she had her band of compatriots. Betty never *relied* on them (or her husbands). They were for companionship and *fun.* They were all playful in different ways.

ONE OF BETTY'S COHORTS WAS A TRUSTED ALLY AND A CHARACTER—Peggy was tall, buxom, and platinum-haired; she would have been cast first as the *heart of gold* who owned the saloon in a classic Old West shoot-'em-up episode. (She reminded me of the pioneer stories of my great-grandmother Zilpha.) There was also Betty's playgirl chum, Caroline, many years younger but the perfect pal with whom to drink, prowl, and hide a couple of decades.

I loved them both, but the friend who had the most influence on me was a Cornell-trained architect a decade older than Betty. Tot was a dignified Eleanor Roosevelt look-alike. In my lifetime, she grew to resemble the bulldogs who were her constant companions. *She grew a studio around a magnificent elm.* In a Frank Lloyd Wrightian approach, she enclosed her brick patio and made a drafting studio. It was stunning to walk inside and feel as if you were outside with the trunk of that elm rising through the roof. It was a rooted, playful, creative chaos of blueprints, books, and *English* Bulldogs.

My first associated memory of her was the immersive experience of a multi-bulldog welcome, which was unforgettable for its drool-baptizing, robust, grunting enthusiasms. Her dogs were always named Butch, Maggie, or perhaps a Beauregard. Tot *got* me. She was *the* reason I found landscape architecture—a career, which was (and is still on occasion) a pretty perfect fit for me.[4]

Betty played in more traditional ways.

"We worked like dogs during tax season, including Pitti-Sing, the cat. We had *fun*." Cindy, one of Betty's young office mates, recounted on a visit from Tulsa.

Pitti-Sing, being a Burmese (and therefore part human and

part monkey), came to the office with Betty each day in their classic gold 280SL Mercedes coupe. Betty barely had to train her; she opened her front door and then the car's door. The cat simply walked out and hopped in to make herself comfortable for the ride to work. They labored long hours from January to Tax Day. At some point in early evening, either Pitti-Sing would get restless and sit on top of the papers that Betty was trying to finish, or she herself would look up and realize the time. Then someone would call out to the others working in the office.

"Do you remember what we used to yell when we had enough?" Leanne asked, the other young office mate of Betty's.

"Bring out the box!" was my mother's quick response. (That would be the gallon box of white wine with a spigot, kept in the fridge…)

My mother knew that *Play Daily* was the long game. My older brother was solidly in this camp: all play, all the time, or so it seemed to me. My mother and he shared that playfulness. She knew how to work hard. She shouldered responsibilities but did not omit the exotic vacations.

However, my ability to play in the trenches (…anywhere but especially in caregiving) was fledgling. Early on, I reached for a dramatic, big playful change—I did Argentinean tango. It was a skill for which I had to take lessons to learn. It required lots of practice, fun black, sexy clothes and late nights out with new tango-dancing girl friends. It was like learning a new language.

The sad and soulful music of the Argentinean bandoneon was the soundtrack to my first six years of caregiving.

WHY DID I RELAPSE INTO WORKAHOLISM? MY OPPORTUNITIES FOR social interactions got smaller, and tango didn't fit the slots. I lost the ability to make better decisions. When you're stuck, it is easy to forget how healing it is to take frequent small social breaks. When I fell ill from the post-traumatic stress of caregiving, and had to get Betty better care in assisted living, I began to stress out in different ways. Instead of focusing on what I could do something about, I saw only Betty's demise creeping up on us, as my bank account edged down.

IN RETROSPECT, ME *PLAYING* WAS ABOUT AS LIKELY AS A DEER-IN-the-headlights completing a math problem—not gonna happen.

Play daily

CAREGIVER STRESS (AND ITS ISOLATION) IS POISON. *PLAY DAILY* IS AN antidote.

Betty's capacity for all things playful was the secret sauce for her long run—our Secretariat race. Finding that lighter moment with friends accessed the good life—*wherever and whenever she was.* She used her time well—moment to moment. She did what she could with what she found—daily. She put little off.

PLAYING IS RESPITE AND RECHARGE.

From the perspective of my own (distant) future hospice bed, all work and too little play looks lame. Take a break—even a small one. Supercharge this remedy *with friends.* Ask them over, telling them to bring a meal (...and a bottle of wine if that works for you).

I LIVED IN A NO-PLAY ZONE MOST OF MY ADULT LIFE.

It is a defensive position that did not move me forward enough for the toll it took so when I became a caregiver, it was a predetermined downward spiral. Deferring gratification in sprints is part of the entrepreneurial dream (which I get) but at some point in the iron-man/woman marathon you gotta call it and let it go. Play daily is part of the healthy caregiving training regime.

PLAYING RIGHT WHERE I AM IS THE LONG GAME—ESPECIALLY IN THE leftover moments.

Integral play is the (new) common sense for uncertain times. It takes faith and bravery to play, trusting that it will all work out. Betty and I found sweetness in the valleys and the vacations. It is the worthiest of efforts to find fun in the middle of the inappropriate, especially, and before it is too late.

7

BE WILLING

IF I AM WILLING, I AM NOT BROKEN.

All the several centenarians that I had the honor of knowing in my caregiving years were playful—in fact they were complete flirts and made fun out of ordinary moments. They helped me in caring for my mother. They were willing to support others—even in their triple numbers. I believe it is how they got to that ripeness. They were willing. No one told them to do it. It just needed doing–and they could.

ALBERTINA X. @ 102

Albertina was only ninety-eight when I met her and she spent her next four birthdays in assisted living with Betty (and me). She sat at my mother's table. She asked for things that Betty forgot she needed. The impish crone was only 102 at the time and famously said, "I am happy to help the old ladies, it is hard when you get to that age." The gentling elder to whom she was referring was my mother at eighty-seven.

ALBERTINA IS A WOMAN WITH A FULL QUIVER OF WIT—BUT UNLIKE

my mother, her zingers didn't draw blood. She is the inverse of my mother—body as tiny and frail as her mind is sharp and robust. She remembers, too. One day, seven years into my caregiving with four to go, she called me on my cell. "I know that Betty is in the hospital and you mentioned that your sweetheart (i.e. my new guy) is out of town. How are you holding up?"

HER COMPASSION *CRUSHED* ME. MY MOTHER HADN'T ASKED ME HOW I was doing for a *decade*. I was alarmed to be so startled—that someone would notice or be curious about me and my inner world. Albertina's warmth showed me my isolation. I was depleted. I started asking for help—or at least I knew that I needed to.

ALBERTINA MAKES IT EASY TO LOVE HER BACK. I WISH I COULD TELL you the story of her wedding cake but she has forbidden it. I think she is being humble, but she might just be kidding me too. If I could tell you, I would take you back to the "Day of Infamy" when not only Pearl Harbor was being bombed but also Hong Kong was invaded. Albertina is a Hong Kong native of Portuguese and Chinese descent. I would tell you how she had to hurry up and get married to her fiancé who had Portuguese citizenship.

"WE NEEDED TO MOVE TO THE SAFETY OF MACAU—IT WAS A neutral state in Portuguese control." Her expression had darkened , "The occupation was very bad," she explained. Clouded by that shadow memory of the unspeakable for a moment, she paused but soon recovered her lightness by telling me this story about her wedding cake. It is a story of how she was loved by her friends—and she still is. It is a story about being willing to caregive each other—in life and death situations.

Her group of friends in Occupied Hong Kong decided that, before she got married, Albertina *must* have a wedding and a cake —despite the Japanese invaders. The wedding was a borrowed affair. Her brother walked her to the church and gave her away because her father was in a Macau refugee camp. "The clothes were easy. There were so many suitcases abandoned on the street from people fleeing the occupation, I had a lot of choices. I was very slim, so I could wear anything." The shoes were harder...she explained, "I have big feet. I had to cut the toes out of the high heels, so I could walk in them."

The cake was even more difficult. Everything was strictly rationed but a few friends divided up the ingredients. Each chum took an illicit ingredient; sugar, flour, eggs, and most important of all was the electricity to bake the cake. "That friend was an engineer, so he knew which power cable to splice."

"If any of my friends were caught by the occupying forces they might have been shot—we didn't think..." She spoke with concern, even seventy years later about the possibly fatal risk they took to bake a cake for her. (She has that effect on people.)

I smiled at her, thinking about the embodied love that cake represented. "Did it taste good?"

Albertina looked at me like she had just remembered, "I never tasted it. It was *too small*. I wrapped up the last piece and saved it for my father to eat when we got to him." A triumphant look overtook her wrinkles, and I could see her as a happy twenty-something offering the precious crumbs to her father once they reached relative safety and reunited in Macau.

For her, it was a tasty bite to remember even at 107. When I asked her about it again, when she herself was in hospice, she was *very* happy that I remembered.

"You're not dead, when someone remembers you."

We remember. Albertina passed away just short of her 108th birthday.

~

Be Willing

If I am willing, *I am not broken.*

How did I find the strength to show up until the end? Being willing was all I had to manage as we inched along.

What do you need to do to *Be Willing* rather than hopelessly overwhelmed? Caregiving can feel like occupied territory. Albertina and other centenarians offer us evergreen examples. They respond to what is in front of them with flexibility and creativity. They solve issues *as they arise,* one by one, and remember what is possible for them to solve. They see and use resources wisely. They watch all that is in motion—circling around them—but remember what is theirs to do with the certainty of a Palu master and an *Etak Compass.*

Love, birth, and death fully unite us as human beings.

The chaos of caregiving is all the same, no matter if I am blue or red, atheist, or evangelical, leftist, progressive, spiritual or whether I believe in evolution, global warming, or not. Grief and loss are intimately woven into our bedside efforts just like leaves fall in their season and new ones grow. Our cells are constantly sloughing off and renewing themselves. I see it as a daily cycle of loss—and renewing life, which everything you see with your eyes and heart is a part of—everything on the planet.

Illness and death closes us down.

If you show up for me, maybe your miserable, flawed, beautiful face is just the thing I need to crack me back open. Every act of affection I have seen or done are breadcrumbs on the path. We caregivers are not alone but accompanied and supported by the seen and the unseen. Every death I have ever attended, or heard, or read about was also a clue. Life grows and dies in such small increments it is hard to see from the ground-truth level any perspective on what is happening or even where I am. It's a garden not a puzzle to be solved.

> "Open your doors."
>
> — NANCY PORTER, MOTHER, SCHOOL TEACHER, SPIRITUAL REFEREE

The lessons from centenarians are about staying open or just re-opening from the constriction of loss. They love who shows up for them.

LOVE WHO SHOWS UP FOR YOU.

> "Show up for death because it teaches you to show up for your life. It is a privilege that does not get an encore."
>
> — MARSHALL WHITE, BETTY'S HOSPICE CHAPLAIN

Show up for the love that loves you back. Be willing. Ask for what you know you need, as it occurs to you. Be kind to yourself.

IF YOU ARE SUPPORTING A CAREGIVER, BE CREATIVE AND FLEXIBLE. Offer specific help, which they are likely to need. Send a card. Be okay with not knowing what to say. Listen. Leave a message. Pay respect (even in a drive-by prayer). Check in. Take time or take food. Show up or just slow down and pay attention.

THE GREATEST SADNESS AT ONE HUNDRED IS THAT MOST EVERYONE you have loved is dead. Centenarians stay alive by being willing to make new friends *among the people who show up for them.* Renewing family, in this way, is a higher order of DNA. Choose well from the people who show up for you, and *Be Willing* to show up for them.

THIS RULE IS RECIPROCAL AND GOLDEN.

If we are willing, we are not broken. We are resilient. In the end, being willing was enough for all the moments, which Betty and I had.

8

STOP. REST.

TAKE OFF YOUR CAPE. DECISIONS WILL BE MADE—BUT NOT RIGHT NOW.

Being willing is usually enough, especially if it is a nap that is required before more Herculean tasks must be performed. Grief is one of those impossibly mythic tasks that humans (eventually) accomplish. In caregiving, grief arrives long before the actual end of life. We *anticipate* it in a million moments, which looks like worry. It takes a toll on us.

WHEN DEATH FINALLY CAUGHT UP TO ME, IT WAS ANTICLIMACTIC and dreamy. In spite of all my efforts and denial of the loss, ('Hey, I already felt *that*...') feelings that still needed to be felt persisted. It seemed to be their mission to do so, and then move on—but only after they have been felt—*to ripeness.* (Incrementally works... the sweet small efforts add up.) The important thing is to be kind to yourself.

WHAT WOULD IT LOOK LIKE IF THE WORLD WANTED YOU HERE?

A few months after my mother passed, I was confronted with the need to caregive myself. Fortunately, my hospice had bereavement counseling available. A few sessions in, I told my new counselor that I was tired and felt deeply overcommitted to caring for others (i.e. the new guy, my old cat, and the people in my life who always *needed* something). I even included him—my counselor. I had clearly demonstrated my distress with him by the indecision of not *leaving* my house *until our appointment time.* It was perhaps our third meeting; I phoned him from my car and started our session on my cell—while driving across the Bay Bridge and into San Francisco to his office, where we finished in person.

He injected these words directly into my earbuds on the drive over, "You are expecting your life to automatically change to what you want overnight. Be gentle. *Rest.* You put your life on hold for eleven years. Give your new life time to unfold."

It was a little alarming how well he listened. He was right. I was not physically tired, as I had just told him. It wasn't that I did *not* want to see him; it was that I did not want to examine my progress or lack of it (on said new life). I also disagreed with him that I had put my life on hold for eleven years. I am a smart woman, why would I do that? If I did, it was not my mother's fault. It was my own fault—if I could not multi-task my life and my mother's life too. *But, wait, what am I saying? That makes no sense.* I ignored the blur of conflicting drive-by thoughts and reported to the counselor...

"I did not make my cash flow goals for this month in my business but I feel like I am making progress. I am not quitting. I am like Edison—I have figured out so many ways that it will not work that I am close to the way it *will* work." I paused mid-report.

I THOUGHT, *BLAH, BLAH, BLAH*...ALL I HEARD FROM MY OWN MOUTH was shaming: *not enough, not enough, not enough.* I stopped talking. This voice—on the phone—my voice, so bores me. *Why is she still here?* I want to slap her—b*ut that would be me, slapping me... not useful.*

SILENCE. I DIDN'T KNOW WHAT TO SAY TO HIM.

MORE SILENCE.

My grief counselor spoke through my earbuds into the empty air space: "What would it look like if the world wanted you here?"

MORE SILENCE.

THE QUESTION WAS LIKE A STUN GUN. *HE'S RIGHT... I HAD NO IDEA...* I teared up. I took a wrong corner; I drove eight blocks in the opposite direction before I got turned around. I was thinking silently of this question, while he waited silently on the other end of the cell for an answer.

BESIEGED IN CAREGIVING FOR SO LONG, I HAD *NO* IDEA WHAT THAT world would look like—the one that wanted *me* here.

Stop. Rest

TAKE OFF YOUR CAPE.

This rule's gentleness hides great power: stop and rest. Caregiving straddles worlds; it is super hero territory. Take off your cape...and take a nap. When it all gets to be too much, I know now, giving myself time to rest is grounding and profoundly compassionate. Listening to myself is necessary to know the next move—the next right step.

It's one of the first questions I ask of caregivers in hospice to assess just how stressed out they are. Even one night's loss of sleep can affect your decisions harmfully—not to mention your immune system.

Decisions will be made—but not right now. We are all carrying a kindness deficit. I am born of the bootstrapped people of the prairie; most of us are sleep-deprived by our ambitions—both thwarted and realized.

Loss of a loved one from dementia is a slow, gradual drip. Though unnamed, I felt the leaching for years long before I became conscious of it. Yet, these incremental losses can reach a tipping point quite suddenly.

Take generous care 'with' yourself. Note, I did not say 'of' yourself (but manicures, hot baths, and Italian underwear are good too). Take generous care *with* yourself, my friends. Rest until you are stronger.

Grief from loss is not purgatory.

It's a womb gestating my inner baritone—the resonating voice of my new life whispering into my earbuds.

II

THE TRENCHES

9

FLASH LIGHT

NAME THE FEAR. IT'S A LIGHT SWITCH— LIGHT ON AND FEAR OFF.

Diva Daughter's Inheritance

It's not like I am a shrinking violet, unable to focus or execute. My friends might say that I am fearless, self-confident, kind, creative, and (a real surprise to me) slightly intimidating.

SEEING THE COMPETENT CAREGIVER, FEW WOULD HAVE GUESSED that I was afraid—most of the time. My anxiety was well hidden and, until recently, unnamed. I osmosed my diva mother's anxiety about the world and have added my own finely tuned "not enoughs." These ideas buzz in the background of my life —like wasps.

MY MOTHER APPEARED FEARLESS. I THOUGHT I WAS THE ONLY ONE who was scared but how could I know what she felt? It isn't as if we *communicated* for the first thirty years of my adult life—unless you count fighting as communication. It got better. I'd like to say we called a détente, but it just happened. Either I was astute enough at being her that she recognized me (her) as acceptable, or I became successful *enough* in the world as a landscape architect that she could relax the mother tiger's hyper-vigilance for fixing her offspring. She wanted to keep me safe and taught me what she knew. She did not intend to teach me fear and insecurity. What she knew was that the corporate world was rigged against people like her (and me). People in power should be looked upon with suspicion. She never actually said this to me. It was woven into the fabric of my pink baby blanket.

Her dementia and death have allowed me to see the story. Here it is—the story I believed without noticing.

Betty valiantly did battle with the world—she was a mythic, exotic, green, dragon queen—capable and crafty. I was the mongrel dragon puppy composed of all soft pink underbelly who just wanted to paint and play in the beautiful weeds.

Since the world so poorly judged the amazing Betty, I feared it would do worse with me.

I thought our fear was courage. I used it to do some of the 'bravest' things in (someone else's) life because I was not so much living my life—but her's. It was so much a part of me that I didn't see. Betty in decline mirrored my own basic assumptions hidden underneath my actions. I realized that being "too soft" was *not* a failing, but the core strength of flexibility. I grew more resilient and mysteriously managed to support Betty to the end of her days, well cared for. That has mattered more to me than anything else.

All in all, I was dealt a privileged hand. Betty got her hand; we all get one. Her decline and death has allowed me to see—some of my core code was malware. I feel the weight of that fear now that my mother has gone. She stored some of it for me, or I held it for her. At her death, I accessed it all for processing.

She gave me the best of what she had.

I own so many gifts from her for a good life, but worry-as-a-worldview is not working (and has never worked well). I choose to let fear die of exposure—in the light.

Flash Light

Every little kid knows what lurks in the dark, under the bed, when the light goes out. It happened to most all of us. When supporting someone you love who's been lassoed by infirmity, the shadows can return quickly when peeking into the great unknowns at the end of life.

It is part of our DNA to scan the horizon for danger; common sense avoids saber tooth tigers. Unfortunately, fear can look useful, seeming to energize us to overcome, but fear defeats us before we start. If my actions are motivated by fear, how successful or happy can I be? It taints all and worse, begets more fear because I am keeping it alive by *living in it.*

WORRY IS THE DIS-EASE OF CAREGIVING. WORRY IS FEAR IN ONE OF its many disguises. It is my reptilian brain firing without any rational explanation. Being hyper-vigilant is fear as a lifestyle choice. Fear pretends to be nuanced but is the same old friend: avoidance of change, dread of illness, or anxiety in making the wrong choice—so I make no choice. Worry is a chameleon. It looks like 'reasonable' planning, but without an action, what's the point?

> "If there is no solution to the problem then don't waste time worrying about it. If there is a solution to the problem then don't waste time worrying about it."
>
> — DALAI LAMA XIV

NAME THE FEAR. IT'S A LIGHT SWITCH—LIGHT ON AND FEAR OFF. (Fireflies do it.) Fear shuts you down. It begins as many things, but in the end *each of them* is dark. What is that but the lack of light? Permeating and disfiguring everything, this fear without a name spoils the quality of moments and blocks me from seeing new possibilities for my life. Without a name, it is amorphous and persistent. Naming it gives you power over the fear. Then you can see clearly what resources you need to deal. It is only one small sweet step to lighting them up.

DO THIS. PROVE IT TO YOURSELF BY SHINING A FLASHLIGHT INTO your night. Watch the shadows run. See for yourself what happens when you do. Name the fear. Flash the light.

I HAVE NO HIGHER GOAL THAN THIS: TO BE LIKE A PRAIRIE FIREFLY.

Shine my own (generated) light into the darkness—I have the power (and the cape). All you need is *enough* light in the dark for the next step—the next right step.

FLASH THE LIGHT. PRACTICE UNTIL YOU KNOW IT IN YOUR BONES. Repeat, as necessary.

10

BOUNCE WELL

BOUNCE IS AN ETHOS...AND CYCLICAL.

Pie Baking Sutras

My grandmother, Annie, was my first example of equanimity. Her world looked broken and she saw wholeness—betting on love and goodness to win over catastrophe. She had some doozies before she was twenty. Her entire generation had a collective case of PTSD. How could they not? The Spanish Flu plague killed fifty million worldwide, WWI slew another seventeen million with twenty million wounded. Then the Depression followed for a decade of deprivation and anxiety. Only my grandmother's divorce deepened her grief to a personal dimension that it was *too much to be felt*—she withdrew from trying romance again, and devoted herself to the household and family.

SHE WAS, NEVERTHELESS, THIS FIRST EXAMPLE OF EQUANIMITY—NOT perfect, and not Buddha-like. Annie's form of it was gracious and generative. It was about survival of *the family.* She did not see healing in the grabbing for *more,* but in supporting others.

She was not Buddha. For one thing, Buddha couldn't bake pies like she could. It was a perfect sutra for kids: the liturgy of comfort food.

Bounce Well

Bounce is an important lesson. Bounce is an ethos.

In the language of the prairie-born, to be "down on your luck" happens to the best of us. To stay there is not just uncomfortable but un-American. The boom and bust economy of my home landscape and the sequential techie bubbles in California are a familiar up and down. You risk, you win (or lose), you are happy (or sad) and you move on to your next best effort. Getting attached to the outcome is neither Buddha-recommended nor is it likely to be useful in caregiving where you can win a few tactical skirmishes, perhaps even a battle or two. The final outcome of the caregiving war *for more time* is beyond our ability to affect.

The notion of *bounce* makes it *cyclical.*

If it is a circle, and if you are still standing, the joy can come round again. Even if it doesn't feel that way, (conceptually) spring *will* follow winter.

My prairie born peeps are neither fragile nor easily broken.

Raised in Oklahoma, I am prairie born and being hardheaded and willful, I know how to endure. My family thrives in disorder and we bounce...*but not all the way back.* We tend not to learn *fully* from the busts, so we are hardly ready for the booms. Dynamic equilibriums are nature's way—swinging, lunging, and balancing

—to move us from one extreme to the other. (It works for healthy grief, too.)

THE DAILY BALANCING SCALES OF SELF-SACRIFICE *AND* SELF-nurture make us resilient.

They also make us ready to bounce with life *as it is—wherever we find ourselves.* Only I can say if I am letting go of that which no longer serves me, or holding on to resentments behind my many masks of fear.

THE *SUSTAINING* LESSONS OF BOUNCE GIVE ME THE FLEXIBILITY TO not go boom in the booms or the extended busts of caregiving.

11

MANGIA, MANGIA

FAST FOOD OR SLOW FOOD, CHOOSE TO MAKE IT REAL FOOD TO FUEL YOUR LIFE.

After working a bust, a boom, and another bust in Tulsa, I signed up for workaholic rehab (i.e. a job) and moved to San Francisco as a Landscape Architect. I only lasted a couple of years as a *payrolled* Landscape Architect, until my next entrepreneurial adventure blossomed with a big-brained programmer husband and our CD-ROM digital atlas company. (It was proto-Googolian with digital maps and aerials synched together before an Internet....or a Google.) As the CEO and Chief Design Officer, I was happy to offload the finances to my mother, who followed me five years later as our CFO. I had no clue that in another five years, it would all implode in the first tech bubble. My caregiving journey of her was a very different kind of bust—it was a shipwreck after a long, long voyage.

During our early caregiving years, my mother and I took several vacations before it became impossible. None were well-advised and all I would do again, if only for the currency of remembered fun, which I can cash just by thinking back.

This next rule offered itself to me after a misadventure with a Mediterranean Sea Captain. (It was not quite the bodice-ripper you are imagining.)

Mangia, Mangia.

Dementia aside, we choose the memories upon which to focus.

Feast and famine, boom and bust, we don't always know from where our next (memorable) meal will come.

> "Life is uncertain; eat dessert first."
>
> — ERNESTINE ULMER, NEBRASKAN AND AUTHOR

My mother repeated this quote so often I thought it original to her.

I want slow savory meals to remember—even if I don't get dessert (or a bodice ripper with a sea captain…). Satisfaction is a good measure of my time on this Earth. As viewed from my future hospice bed, even an unrequited pull of the red ribbon (…that would be my halter top in a girlQuantum story of a cruise out of Venice) is a memory that entertains, if not nourishes.

I hope to be tasting the pleasures of *real foods* until the end —especially the ones that sustain and spark me. Perhaps the menu of caregiving 'responsible' choices du jour dictate that I skip a few meals, but won't that make the next one even more pleasurable?

> "Hunger is the best sauce."
>
> — CICERO IN DE FINIBUS (ON THE ENDS OF GOOD AND EVIL)

Fast food or slow food, I choose to make it real food.

You are what you eat, *so I choose to consume more love,* thank you very much. Is there love in my love? Is there love in your meals?

MANGIA, MANGIA IS THE WAY MY ITALIAN, HEARTH-MAKING grandmothers *say it.*

Take it in. Digest your worthiness in every mother of a mitochondria you have. Give yourself the gift of authenticity: listen to your longings and discontents. They are navigation to a life well lived.

CHOOSE THE GOOD FOOD THAT BEST FUELS *YOUR* LIFE.

12

BEDROCK ALLOWING

ALLOW THE 'IMPERFECT' IN. IT MAY, GIVEN A CHANCE, APPRECIATE YOU BACK.

As much as a full belly of good food (or good words) satisfies, some emptiness is beyond even a good meal. Caregiving comes to mind.

IN THE BEGINNING, IT WAS ALL SO CLEAR. I KNEW WHAT TO DO: *TAKE her to the ER and have them fix her.* Dementia started obscuring Betty soon after the bankruptcy of our digital atlas company and my brother's death, but I could still reach the 'old Betty' who I remembered, especially if we were planning a party or a trip.

FOR OUR LAST VACATION TOGETHER, THE CHRISTMAS MARKETS OF the Rhine, I am three and a half years into caregiving with seven more to go and then another in hospice. I am mid-lesson and in process of learning a deepening compassion for my mother—and for myself too. It is a puzzle with *only me* as the confused puzzle-master—still in the purgatory of making increasingly ineffective attempts to *make* her well; I am feeling the stress of being the sole administrator of our lives.

I REPEAT EVERYTHING TWENTY TIMES; SHE FORGETS. THE repetition wears me down; she is not a child. She *does not learn.* I mistakenly see who she *used* to be, the capable mother, not the child-in-mother's-clothing she is now. I need to retire my habit of making this about Betty's failures or blaming something (or someone) for my conundrum—but I am stuck *here.*

ONE MORE TIME...

She is smaller now...and sweeter.

SHE SAYS SHE APPRECIATES ME. THIS IS A *GOOD* THING. IT FEELS healing, but then I succumb to my own inclement weather and I think I am merely useful to her.

THERE ARE FEWER OF THOSE DAYS NOW. IT TAKES TOO MUCH ENERGY for that kind of doublethink drama. It is uselessly circular; I am moving but it's not getting me anywhere I want to go.

THIS MID-CAREGIVING SNAPSHOT OF BETTY IS THROUGH THE aperture of my own fatigue. It is through this sad lens that I offer this rule...

OKAY, HERE IT IS: I *CAN* CHOOSE TO RUN...BUT I WILL NEVER BE able to reach escape velocity from 'what is." I cannot change *this.* I must caregive 'what is.' This rule is about not resisting but allowing 'what is'...*in*.

Bedrock Allowing

I MUST FIGURE OUT HOW TO LOVE THE UNLOVABLE—THE WEAK, THE fragile, and *the crepey.*

I must caregive 'what is. Up to that point, I was *so sure* of the *structure* of my life. My mother would rally. She always had. It was *understood.* That scaffolding was my self-protection. I relied on it, and her. However, when faced with my mother's implosion on our riverboat vacation, my ground truth cracked with her.

WHO COULD BE SO DELUSIONAL TO THINK THAT DEATH AND DECLINE would never come to them? Most of us do, until we can no longer hold that worldview to be plausible. (Only then do we sign our advanced directives...)

THERE WAS NOWHERE TO RUN ON THAT RIVERBOAT. LOVE MADE ME caregive 'what is'.

I found myself tight into a corner, which *required* of me a deep surrender. My own soft flesh mirrored hers. Even as I have had considerable compassion for Betty, I had not extended the kindness to myself. (Who me? Needy and weak? *Never...*) But if *Betty* could so fail, I was logically next. It was so much easier for me to accept decline *in her*—because it wasn't me—but this caregiving of her became the practice of acceptance, and allowing, and kindness *for me*.

IN DOING THIS, I RECEIVED A REVELATION—A SORT OF ONENESS BY shotgun.

There was a clarity of distance. I became a witness. I was a watcher...watching my mother move ever closer to the *Maker of All Things*—and here I was right behind her.

OUCH AND—AWESOME...

It was good to find bedrock. Allowing and accepting myself, or you, 'as is' frees *me*.

ALCOHOLICS IN AA, ALL HAVE THEIR 'BOTTOM' STORIES—THEIR worst remembrance.

This trip down the Rhine was my bottom—my "valley of the shadow." I was depleted. Betty wouldn't come out of our riverboat's cabin *and was happy about it.* I took her meals to her and was alone, at the holidays, with a bunch of strangers, who pitied me. I should have been seeing cheery red and green decorations at Christmas markets, but all I saw was the blue of the snow, the people and my mood.

YET, I DISCOVERED BEDROCK—THE SOLID EARTH UNDER OUR FROZEN turbulence. There I found the principle to see the *true nature of the* gifts waiting for me in the dark, under my own skin. *It was a complete reset of my cultural operating system.*

ALL STRUCTURES ARE UNSTABLE BUT I HAVE RICH *INTERIOR resources...and the choice of how I see*. Blessed are those who hunger and thirst for we tend to look past appearances—toothless, overstuffed, or bungled up and in pieces. They may be *more than enough* to ease and heal...if I allow them in.

I RETURNED TO SAN FRANCISCO WITH AN EXHAUSTED MOTHER AND other *very heavy* baggage.

We were met at the airport by a couple of friends who had known their own crumbling structures. They both had more than a few *dead in their heads,* too. One was a neighbor who was taking care of our house and cats, the other, a business partner. We were greeted with a ride from the airport, flowers, help with the luggage, and dinner in the refrigerator. I was not expecting that gift, but needed it. It was sustaining.

TAKE OFF YOUR CAPE AND HOLD OUT YOUR HANDS.

Remembering this renews my gratitude and confirms that I was *not* alone even when I most felt that I was. I had help. You do too. Allow it in.

ALLOW THE 'IMPERFECT' IN. IT MAY, GIVEN A CHANCE, APPRECIATE you back.

Gifts still come to me more frequently than I can accept, but I *see* them now. That is the Rx for a *sustainably* good life. The practice of *Bedrock Allowing* is a core skill for a renewable life.

13

LEAN BACK

LEAN BACK INTO WAITING ARMS—SEE WHO IS STILL THERE WHEN YOU DO.

Not being clear what a normal childhood is, I am fairly sure that I didn't have one. *Bedrock Allowing* is, in any case, both strategic and tactically useful in saving time on weepy *what-ifs* about *what-never-was.*

No doubt I inherited sustaining stories from my great-grandparents (GGs), grandparents (Gs), four fathers (there were four of them), and Betty, but this is real life. Some stories, if they ever worked, no longer did. Others were buggy. The businesses and crops I thought I planted didn't fruit (or got gobbled up by pests). Other things sprouted—without asking me for permission. Caregiving of my mother for eleven years was *not* in my plans.

Betty Did Not Ask

Generosity was my mother's M.O. Her example showed me how to live and give but not to ask. Asking was my lesson from caregiving and one of the best things about my new story. As her daughter, I got good at guessing what was going on—much of caregiving is like that. Guesstimating is good; intuiting is useful. However, making stuff up is dangerous. I have lost myself (and a marriage) in my personal mythic tales that may or may not have ever been true. It is easy to do if your stories are a way to make sense of what you don't understand, or about people who won't say, or tend to sulk. (Yep…thinking about the ex.)

It's a beautiful gift when people tell you what's going on with them. It's the best present.

The endurance battle to care for my mother cured me of most of the nonsense of not asking for help when I need it. I became so depleted and exhausted emotionally and financially that by year nine, I just started asking. It was more like a drowning man's grab than any reasonably framed adult query, but I began to learn a better way.

The Benefits of Asking

People showed up when we needed them. Sometimes I asked, and sometimes it took just *being willing* to be helped for them to find us. My new friends might be ephemeral or lifelong. A flow of kindnesses sustained us. There wasn't one teat reserved for us on the providential udder, we were fed by many.

Here are two bracketing paper-doll angel events from the first half of our caregiving years:

The first was serendipitous support. Freshly into my first year of caregiving, ignited by my brother's fall from the sky (death by skydiving), and gut-punched by Betty's half dozen ER visits, we seemed to have reached the far shore. Unaware it was only a tiny island in an eleven-year archipelago, we chose North Beach for dinner. I could see Betty was tender, but I savored the flavor of our connection in our meal all evening. It wasn't just the Venetian-Hungarian, woman-chef at the restaurant, or the old-world homespun charm of their Craigslist collection of glass tables, iron chairs, and dishware. It was our own intimate connection back to those regular Monday lunches as peers back in Tulsa where the restaurant staff knew us well. In *my* plans, this eatery was to be our new hangout in North Beach. Its immigrant proprietors seemed to appreciate the linkage of femme family. Maybe, our mother-daughter, living-DNA, time-lapse cameos evoked their own internal mamma-memories but they seemed to love us back. However it happened, we ate joy in that food. (*Mangia, Mangia,* indeed).

On the way back, feeling happy and grateful, walking arm in arm the long two blocks back to the apartment, Betty shut down. Her knees buckled and I was left holding all her weight with both my hands.

"Should I call an ambulance, honey?" Looking around for a door to knock on, to raise some stranger with a 911 landline. (It is so easy to forget a pre-cellular world.) Betty adamantly refused.

"No, not now...not again. Please, get me to bed. That's all I need." I started moving *but she didn't.* I stood there stuck, unable to shift her. Putting her down on the pavement would mean I would have to pick her up again—a disastrous option.

That was what the two young women saw as they turned the corner. They were having their own jovial evening, laughing and chatting.

I asked for help.

The paper-doll angels accordioned themselves to either side of Betty, walking her the half block ahead of me while I fumbled for the keys to the apartment. The stellar view of North Beach (with all the stairs it necessitated) seemed like the inanest idea I had ever had, but to those two steppers, steps weren't a problem. Betty was into bed, and they let themselves out before I could thank them.

I wish I had thanked them, then. I hope they knew.

No...let me thank them, now. "Wherever you two are, may you receive as graciously as you gave, and may help be given freely when you *need* it most.

The second paper-doll angel event occurred five more years into her dementia and six before Betty died.

It was a beautiful afternoon when Betty touched the ocean for the last time. A few months later, she would fall and be prescribed assisted living. The unavoidable truth was that she was no longer a one-daughter task; her instability required more than twenty-four/seven of me.

A COUPLE OF MY FRIENDS HAD SHOWN UP TO HELP ME GET HER OUT of the apartment for the afternoon. We went to Beach Chalet near Ocean Beach in San Francisco for lunch.

SHE AND I HAD JUST COME FROM THE RESTROOM; I WAS DISTRACTED, disconcerted and thinking. *My mother is no longer potty-trained... and it does not bother her...she seems so happy.* (Toilet details will be spared.)

I WAS IN THE PROCESS OF, INEFFECTIVELY, PUTTING A HAPPY FACE ON mine, when the mural images of several women on the lobby's walls compelled me. A plaque immortalized the long dead, fresco artist Lucien Labaudt. It was one of the public works of art rendered by the Depression's unemployed via the Works Progress Administration. The world needed strong women to survive plague, war, Depression, and another war that had to be won. I was transported by the durable beauty of these women who were painted in 1936: young, hearty, and healthy. They *were Betty's cohorts.* Their health held me for a long moment. I envied their evergreenness, and wondered if their daughters were as stuck as I was.

I TURNED TO FIND MY MOTHER. SHE AND OUR COMPANIONS WERE gone. After a typical caregiver panic attack and search, I saw them.

My two friends, a woman, pushing 6'1" and the man, a real giant, at 6'4", were walking Betty out across a football field of sand to touch the surf *because she asked to go.* I watched their silhouettes against the early sunset like two oversized paper cutout figures holding a smaller (and smaller) doll between them. Betty was happy like a puppy in those four big, capable, *and kind* hands. Love was in motion—to the edge of the continent and back. Both friends fell out of my life soon after this but the waves of immense gratitude still flow for them. Their paper-doll angel accordion enveloped me just after I realized my need, but before I had to humble myself to ask. Their acts of kindness remain with me, and now with you.

Coinage and Currency

When I finally started asking, *because I had to,* I began to understand that asking is the flip side of giving. Until the money ran out in caregiving, I had an imperfect understanding of giving, too. I was generous in giving but all dried up at the receiving. Life continues to give me practice with these currency and checkbook basics—and it's not about the money (but it's that, too).

Asking is the coin. Giving and receiving are its two sides. This asking-needing-receiving thing... is connected. I found this place when caregiving Betty and I believe she did too—this place of connectedness and currency where who is giving and who is receiving is blended into one thing. It's inconvenient and it's love in motion.

Like a Mobius, the international recycling symbol, its path only *appears* to have two independent sides. (Imagine a short length of ribbon. Before you connect one end to the other, give it a half twist...) As you trace your finger along the ribbon of a Mobius strip, you understand it has *just one side—just one journey.* There is a point in caregiving where it is hard to tell the difference between who's receiving and who's giving. I listen to the story, which you *need* to tell, and it may be exactly the idea or notion that guides me in my next right step out of my stuckness.

I FIND IT DAILY AS MY PATIENTS TEACH ME ABOUT THE COURAGE IT takes to live. It is gratifying to support them—to be allowed to do it.

I SEE FROM HERE A HUMANITY AND HUMILITY IN LOSS—AND IN asking for help—but if my giving is your recycled ask, the whole picture offers up a flow of gratitude in a kinder world. Compassion and interconnectedness is the coin of this realm. Until *I had to* ask, I did not understand what a privilege it is for me to respond to *your* request. It is my gift of *need to them and their gift to respond.* No flip of the coin is possible in this quantum universe. There is no *other* side.

ASKING ALSO ASSUMES I AM WORTHY OF A YES. IT'S THE BUBBLES, and busts of life that make it renewable.

IF YOU HAVE A HISTORY OF GENEROSITY BUT NO UNDERSTANDING OF our common fragility, by never having had the *karmic* tables turned on you, *you may miss it.* It means being supported when you need it. We are all part of this human family, and family helps family. You don't know who is behind you in life's tender valleys until you look back...or lean back into waiting arms. The gift that my grandmother knew but my mother missed is the understanding that it is all a gift.

~

Lean Back

I LEARNED RESILIENCE IN THE UPS AND DOWNS (ECONOMIC AND emotionally) of Tulsa. The flatland economy is built on booms and busts so there is a lot of individual experience with bouncing and splatting. Giving is easier than asking. *Lean Back* is one of the renewable lessons—the centenarians know. If you are willing to show up in the busts of others, you are more likely to find people who will show up *for you*. *Be Willing* to receive is the durable way to renew your life. These are the inherent checks and balances in the booms and busts.

> "Out of clutter, find simplicity. Out of discord, find harmony. In times of difficulty find opportunity."
>
> — ALBERT EINSTEIN

I WAS NOT TAUGHT TO ASK. ASKING SHOWED YOU WERE WEAK.

THE MORE EVERGREEN PRAIRIE LESSON IS ABOUT NEIGHBORLINESS and community. You are superbly blessed if you have a *DNA family* (or perhaps it is found family) *who gets you*—DNA of the heart. The living fabric of support is *interdependence; it is sustainable power of woven living light*—even if I am too dark, on occasion, to see it. Being solidly in community means that I am more likely to find help because the current is flowing throughout the network.

I give myself permission to be a part of this Earthly commons, by asking.

Since it is not easy to ask for help, (maybe it shouldn't ever be easy to ask...) it gives me the opportunity to clarify what I need. My asking may even help others by being an example of how to ask with grace and the *lack of any shame.* It gives others permission to be connected. It is the basis of our commons.

Asking is courageous. Like blood, money needs to circulate to be healthy.

It's like inhaling and exhaling. Ask. Give. Receive. Celebrate your time here with others. It's love in motion—it's improv. It's also possible your people will be AWOL when you need them. People are not always loving, loyal, and kind. It happens.

Lean back into waiting arms—see who is still there when you do.

If those connections are *not* there, pick yourself up, and be grateful for the clarity—it's the feedback that feeds you. It's *Feed Me Feedback.* Go find better friends. *Be one.*

For this reason, I recommend a test lean *before* a crisis. Asking threshes out the keepers. Be a keeper *to* yourself.

14

IT TAKES AS LONG AS IT TAKES

GRIT IS INSANELY USEFUL IN CAREGIVING, BUT IN GRIEF—NOT SO MUCH.

After my mother passed, there was no *Lean Back.* More like flat on my back, I greyed-out for a time. Trying hard not to fade with her, a dreamy unreality confined me in a sort of bubble prison. Colors in my world parched out into a desert *lightness,* which made me more tired and *thirsty.* I felt like the dusty potted plant in the corner silently screaming for water as a peopled office took breaks at the water cooler.

THIS SHRIVELED PROVIDENCE OF LOSS LANDED ME IN A GRIEF GROUP and it took time to unravel us.

It Takes as Long as it Takes

BEING FROM THE AMERICAN PRAIRIE WITH OUR OVERDEVELOPED work ethic, we don't *do* grief but force ourselves up and onward. However, this self-denial is not unique to the prairie. It happens with many—especially fresh emigrants. They work hard and ache to feel (again) a safety of *belonging*.

WORKING HARD AT GRIEF DOESN'T WORK. I MUST *ALLOW* IT TO work me.

A 'NORMAL' BEREAVEMENT IS ALWAYS *TOO* LONG... IF YOU ARE mourning, it's healthy to dwell (even wallow...), so when ready you can move forward, ripe to begin life again. If we have mourned the loss, to keep moving optimistically makes a lot of living sense. The trouble is, when life inevitably brings us to our knees, my people—those from the prairie—do not generally stay down long enough to feel what needs to be felt. We don't dwell long enough to heal our resilience—or I didn't.

GRIT IS INSANELY USEFUL IN CAREGIVING, BUT IN GRIEF—NOT so much.

IF I DON'T PROCESS THIS LOSS NOW, IT WILL FOLLOW ME, FOR YEARS. Frankly, I don't have that kind of time. I don't want to ski past or parachute over it; I want to parse the passings of my mother (and most of my family) because deferred and denied grief does not scale. Something in me died with Betty but something else is growing—seeds are germinating in this darkness, waiting until conditions are right (and ripe).

> "For even as love crowns you so shall he crucify you. Even as he is for your growth so is he for your

> pruning. Even as he ascends to your height…so shall he descend to your roots and shake them in their clinging to the earth."
>
> — KAHLIL GIBRAN, THE PROPHET

GRIEF DOES SOME PRUNING. YOU CAN DO A LOT OF DAMAGE TO THE structure of a tree (or a human) if you don't consider the pruning. If I do grief well, the dead wood gives way to stronger branching and a more vigorous life. Unlike an actual tree, the metaphor is wilier. Though I would like this grief to end, I want it done well and that *takes as long as it takes.*

LISTEN TO YOUR OWN CLOCK.

IGNORE THE CULTURAL TIMEKEEPERS WHO ARE ALL TOO HAPPY TO tell you what, how much and how long grief will take. Err on the side of kindness for yourself and your new life. If I am kind, pain will not become suffering. *You* will know when it is time to move on. Yes, you may linger a bit longer than necessary or optimally efficient. Wallow away.

I NEED TO LET MYSELF SLOW. *STOP. REST…*UNTIL I AM DONE WITH it. Marinate in the loss until you are sick of it. It may be the quickest way to get ready to let *them* honorably go. Grief is the backside of love; it's what love looks like when we begin to know (or even suspect) our loss. Honor your love by feeling it fully because love can take it. It is a superpower of holding opposites.

Grow something wonderful in your tilled soil of loss. The next best chapter of my life waits on this investment of time in the trenches of love.

15

KEEP MOVING

ALLOW PROVIDENCE TO FLOW TO YOU AND THROUGH YOU. TAKE THE NEXT STEP, EVEN IF SMALL.

The long valleys of loss take time to navigate. Finding a hardy, loving few standing with you to listen and break bread with is a great gift. It is a one of the blessings of illness, caregiving, and grief to see the warp and weave of our connections. Our repair may then progress in the telling (and re-telling) of our stories.

Obstacles to the Good Life

My mother explained the navigation of life to me this way. "I was walking to work on Market Street one morning while working in San Francisco just after the war. (That would be WWII.) I had on a suit jacket and a wide skirt in the style of the late forties." She confided to me that her silk undershorts were a recent extravagance and reward to herself—she was an early adopter of retail therapy. They were loose and silky, fastened at the waist with only one slim mother-of-pearl button. "While I was walking, I felt that button pop off." She paused. "Those shorts slid down my legs right there with so many people walking by. Without missing a step, I stopped and picked them up..." She then demonstrated to me the lady-like, delicate manner with which she bent at the knee, seized them, "...and I kept walking."

THAT WAS THE WAY WE WERE *SUPPOSED* TO DEAL WITH OBSTACLES—keep moving.

ELIZABETH (OR AS I CALLED HER BETTY) WAS ALWAYS IN MOTION—going to work or some well-behaved, old-school Republican soirée. However, once the doors of commerce (of whatever serial CPA partnership with which she was involved at that point) had closed at the end of the day, she danced a more socially liberal step. I learned all her tricks, sometimes by apostolic transmission, sometimes by direct instruction. My mother explained the issues and opportunities blocking her as a woman this way:

"GET OVER IT." SHE WAS EMPHATIC AND EXHALED THE WORDS WITH a deep impatience. It was the first message I remember about the operating instructions of her world; I knew it was very, very important but I was not sure what she meant. I might have been ten at the time.

HOLY INDIGESTION

With the death of my mother, the last layer of generational "protection" is gone. Now I am digesting it all by myself and all these voices are upsetting.

EVEN IF THEY WERE ONLY EPHEMERAL AND ILLUSORY, THESE LAYERS

were friendly, familiar, and blocked a dangerous world's access. I was a good daughter. That identity had meaning for me in the world—or it did.

WHO AM I NOW? WITH MY OLDER BROTHER DEAD, I AM NO LONGER a middle child, I am now the *eldest.* All protective layers of fathers and mothers are gone, too; the little family I have left is very far away. I also feel the weight, too, of the family that I did not make —no children of my own. The gravity of this makes me not recognize the reasoning within my own incremental milestones and decisions. Hey—these things happen; it's life. I make choices in the moment. I play hunches and hope they are reasonable. The gamble works out, or it doesn't. I placed well behaved, "good girl" bets: I chose a big-brained programmer to husband me; he promised forever and then just...changed his mind—eleven years later. Life happens.

STAKING YOUR SAVINGS ON A BUSINESS IS NO DIFFERENT. IT MIGHT do well, or it might fail. Venture capitalists herd together to diversify their risk, share and reinforce memes, and then hope that, perhaps, a tenth of their contenders will be successful. This would be a rotten average, if they weren't betting in the big time. Like them, we are all wishing to get hit with the golden shrapnel in the next big disruptor product explosion (not the bubble's inevitable implosion). Or maybe, like Betty, you place your bets closer to home. She bet on the next husband, tax season, vacation, or beautiful thing. Prairie lessons are *all about* boom and bust. Flatland mettle is not suppressed for long.

YOU WIN SOME, YOU FAIL AT OTHERS.

"So? Let's go." I can hear the voice of my mother saying this from behind me. She is (even dead and only in my memory…) quick to get over things. I process longer, (or just that I *do* process). "What are you saying, daughter…that I am shallow or don't think things through?" The more I listen to her voice, the more she speaks to me but she is only *playing* petulant...

I answer her, out of a sense of therapeutic play. "No, honey. I don't have insight into you and how you made the decisions you did." *(Just that you were mercurial compared to me.)* I feel uncomfortably naked right now admitting these vulnerabilities (*I hear dead people...)* but I refuse to edit them out. Grief is so tightly cyclical. It shuts me down. It has again violently unearthed my most persistent question: Who can I trust now to help me? Who is my team? How can I get support? Who can I trust to *be* there when I need them, when most of my people are dead?

"You are a *terrible* judge of character." My (remembered) Betty is not playing around now. She is frustrated that I am showing weakness to the world. She taught me better.

Suddenly, I am eight, again. (Grief is awful; I feel pathetic and confused.) Her voice is so clear…and loud, but, hey, if it was true then, it is not true *now. "Thanks for sharing, darling. Aren't you due to go have lunch with John W. right now?"* I try to distract her.

Starting again from right where I am is healing—even though it looks awkward and lame. I want to move but am stuck here. All I can do is repeat the rule so many times that it is tattooed on the *inside* of my forehead:

It Takes as Long as it Takes...
It Takes as Long as it Takes...
It Takes as Long as it Takes.

I NEED A PATIENT, BARITONE VOICE TO HELP ME BECAUSE MY OWN voice is saying, "Get over it" (which is not kind). Even though slow, or only able to take baby steps, or even two steps forward, one back, even when pausing to *Stop. Rest* or *Wait Here, I am moving.*

Keep Moving

I MET AN AMAZING WOMAN AT HER HUNDREDTH BIRTHDAY PARTY—Grandma Olga.

She sparkled with gravitas; it was not just her eyes but also her countenance. She had come over on the boat from Prague to America as an adolescent. Since then she had married, had lots of children, lived through hard times, and good times. She was now surrounded by grandkids, and many great, great (great) relationships.

"WHAT IS YOUR SECRET?"

I asked her in the middle of the happy chaos. She answered in the grounded way that only a vintage old woman with deep roots and healed scars can. She looked me in the eye and said: *"Keep moving."*

"LET'S GO."

I hear a voice behind me that sounds just like my mother (but it is all me now) trusting my gut to deal with whatever life brings. 'We' now have an understanding to digest the world *together*—separating the useful stuff from the BS. We have everything we need *to keep it moving.*

> "It is the same with people as it is with riding a bike. Only when moving can one comfortably maintain one's balance."
>
> —ALBERT EINSTEIN, IN A LETTER TO HIS SON, EDUARD 1930

Take big bites of life and *savor the chewing*. Take the next step, even if small. Stuckness is the eternal disease of being afraid. Keep moving toward healing—especially in the small courageous (and kind) acts. Consider letting go of the notion that you *have* control in the first place.

ALLOW PROVIDENCE TO FLOW TO YOU AND THROUGH YOU. HOLDING on to nothing, but trusting your belly to digest it all—the sweetness, the nutrients and the junk-food judgments. It's love working its way through the world. The remaining indigestible BS goes back to the good Earth from which it came.

16

DO BOTHER

WOVEN UNDER THE SURFACE OF THINGS, LOVE WANTS TO BE BOTHERED WITH YOUR TROUBLES.

The edges of our caregiving stories are messier in real time than in retellings. We need to tell and retell our stories over and over—to keep it moving and to make it real. We are all just sleepwalkers until we do because the loitering proximity of death, changes your viewpoint; it's an otherworldly wake up call for even the most habitual 'hit-the-snooze-button-again' aficionados. People think differently—after.

GRIEF IS A HARROWING AND NEVER A FUN PARTY COMPANION—NOR is it dating talk. Yet, halfway into my caregiving decade, the soon-to-be new guy came back after I cancelled our first date in lieu of my own visit to the ER. I was so stressed by five years of caregiving that I developed a hole in my stomach from the overwhelm and was bleeding internally. I ignored it until I collapsed. It was not a coincidence that *my own* hospital stay corresponded with one of Betty's (in a different hospital) and her subsequent assisted living RX. I couldn't do it anymore alone.

THE GUY BROUGHT ME FLOWERS *IN THE HOSPITAL.* (WHO DOES that?) I met him at my church; he was nice, which had been the disconnect signal in my early life, but I let him in. He wore me down with his persistence—and his flowers. Our (*second*) first date was dinner, which was close enough to Valentine's Day, that he brought me two dozen red roses... *and chocolate.*

"TOO MUCH?" HE ASKED ME AS HE HANDED ME THE ROSES AND candy at the door. What could I do but lie? It was only polite...

WE GOT THROUGH IT, SOMEHOW. IT WAS GRACE.

WE WERE WILLING TO BE BOTHERED.

Do Bother

IT'S OKAY THAT YOU ARE A BOTHER. I AM, TOO. *BOTHER ME.* SPEAK. Don't spare me. Show me what you need. I will respond if I am able.

LOVE FOR THE LONG HAUL MATERIALIZES IN ACTS OF SERVICE. IT IS the kind of love that is creative. (We shelter each other to form community.) This love hangs around—and it's a bother. Vulnerability and reciprocal growth of trust are the secrets to its strength and sustainability.

WOVEN UNDER THE SURFACE OF THINGS, LOVE *WANTS* TO BE

bothered with your troubles. Betty did not teach me this kind of love. She knew about it, but didn't value it. Annie, my grandmother, did.

I NEED THIS KIND OF LOVE NOW—IN THE CAREGIVING OF MY good life.

17

CACKLE

CALL UP THE "EVIL" QUEEN (IN YOUR GRIEVANCE STORY DU JOUR). SAY YOU'RE BUYING DINNER.

My prairie roots know about bothering with family and friends; it is caregiving 101 and how they survived. They did it together, but when death killed off the good stewards in my familial bloodline, fear became the cultural operating system in my life.

I HOLD BOTH OF THESE: MY MOTHER, BETTY, WAS BRAVE IN THE world; she showed generosity and great style but she was a not a warm and tender mommy figure. She loved me but did a not-too-terrific job of showing me. She threw me scraps of time and left me wanting more of her. How could she do otherwise? Betty was thrown scraps, too. Her father (who was her hero) multi-tasked his love. Upon who could she pattern her life if not her heroes?

APPARENTLY, BETTY AND I ARE PART OF THE HUMAN FAMILY, surrendering to (or resenting) the imperfect love that comes our way. Cackle is about a forgiving attitude; it is not an event. I hear forgiveness in my mother's laughter now and every time I, myself, laugh deeply. Her's is so throaty, she outright cackles. It is beautiful—and contagious.

CACKLE IS *NEVER* A COMPLIMENT TO A WOMAN; IT IS *NOT* 'LADY-LIKE' laughter. A man guffaws; he roars, chortles, belly laughs but he does not cackle. Like bitch, it tends to be a woman-only shaming word; it's always associated with someone *else's* old woman, or one who is *not* from *your* community. The belly laugh of *your old lady,* granny, mommy, or auntie is *heartwarming*. This rule is about grounding into the unknowing and (as Rumi says) befriending bewilderment. We cannot know or control it all—or much (besides our attitude).

IT IS ABOUT EMBRACING UNCERTAINTY—JOYFULLY AND WITH friends.

Cackle

CACKLE IS ANTI-DELUSIONAL BECAUSE IT RECOGNIZES THAT WE don't know (and don't control) much.

ALL HUMAN INNOVATION IS ABOUT MAKING SOMETHING different...and better. Betty wanted a different life than that of her foremothers. She chose a very different path from her peers. Who knows *in the trenches of creation* what the outcome of our decisions (or delusions) will be over time?

DIFFERENT MIGHT *BE* BETTER—OR, POSSIBLY, DISASTER. WE GATHER data, research known facts, do opinion surveys, but it's all just a weather report filtered through the cultural corsets *du jour.* We find out by playing it out. We find out by doing it anyway. At worst, we will have eliminated a regret at the end of life, or perhaps, played out a better probability. We may even evolve—it's no sure thing.

CACKLE IS ABOUT DOING IT ANYWAY

CACKLE IS A POWERFUL RULE BECAUSE IT INFERS THE ROAD-TESTED (but still mysterious) wisdom of letting go of the outcome. There is a non-obvious courage innate in this rule. It is about doing the next right thing, no matter the worries in my recipe of decision-making ingredients.

I AM RETICENT TO QUOTE THE WISDOM OF MY GRANDFATHER BUT HIS adage is wise in the scheme of wanting different: "Do something, damn it, even if it is wrong." It has courage–especially when we are stuck not knowing which way or what to do next. At some point, we must step out in faith toward something or someone—maybe even ourselves.

CACKLE HELPS YOU STEP OUT WITH A LITTLE SEED OF FAITH *IN yourself* for your *next* right step. Cackle is about planting and tending your seeds even if you find yourself watering them on the edge of the known, in the Biblical wilderness, where we have forgotten who we are.

YESTERDAY, I VISITED ALBERTINA. SHE IS 107, IN HOSPICE AND living on the love of (and for) her visitors and family. I sat with her and (mostly) listened for a couple of hours. She complained about God that afternoon. She was still having a lover's quarrel with Him...for his very poor worldly management skills and the uneven care at her assisted living facility. I listened and mirrored what she was saying to let her know she was heard. (Such are the superpowers of a friend.) She was laughing so hard when I left, at herself and the world that she cried. She got there by herself but I shared the moment with her. Her face was practically skeletal at this point—*and so lovely.*

> "The human race has only one really effective weapon and that is laughter.
>
> — MARK TWAIN

IF ANNE LAMOTT COULD HAVE SEEN ALBERTINA'S FACE JUST THEN, she would have seen a 'carbonated holiness' there. Albertina forgave God that afternoon for his mismanagement, and simply bubbled up with what was right in front of her—*even confined to her bed.* She was effervescent.

CACKLING IS ABOUT INVITING IN THE HAPPY MOMENT—TOGETHER with found family (or whoever shows up in love). *Be Willing* is that renewable centenarian rule about making community with people who are *reciprocal* in relationship—allowing love to show up for you by how you show up for love.

CALL UP THE "EVIL" QUEEN (IN YOUR GRIEVANCE STORY DU JOUR). Say you're buying dinner. Laugh until you're both snorting.

I AM ON THE HUNT FOR MORE AND SUSTAINABLE JOY. AT THIS POINT, gratefully, I know it hides everywhere (in the mitochondria of being)...but it's a cosmic crapshoot *to find it from my unknown.*

A JOYFUL CACKLE WITH FRIENDS IS THE BEST OF NAVIGATORS.

18

PHOENIX CAROUSEL

INSPIRE A RENEWAL—LIGHT THE MATCH. EVEN IF YOU THINK IT'S YOUR LAST ONE.

Caregiving is seldom funny and consistently challenging. Sometimes, the best defense (and the bravest thing I can do) is to grin at the chaos—a *Cackle* would be even better. It's about remembering in the trenches about the hum of a happy universe—or possibly a vacation.

Vacations to Come

As scavengers of a former life, Betty and I set about looking for new ones. Parts of that search turned into four vacations—none of them wise. All were beyond Betty's physical ability and my own probabilities of relaxation. After that, traveling for her meant time-travel where the only way to accompany her was quantum.

"Let's go." I remember my mother saying. My friends thought I was nuts.

TRAVELING IS THE OPPORTUNITY FOR BIG CHUNKS OF *MEMORABLE* play. The trips with Betty and family make me happy even now—just remembering. They generate gratitude. Vacations are important but does it make any sense at all to only play *two weeks* out of your entire year?

WHAT WOULD BETTY SAY? (WWBS?) *"LET'S GO." (IT WAS HER unofficial mantra.)*

LA BEFANA'S STORY—SANTA AS AN OLD WOMAN

The Italian New Year was a panoply of perfect distractions (all edible by mouth or eye)—the pasta, the prosciutto, the panna cotta, and the lights were everywhere. It was a broth of reduced and savory stock with the most delicious that humanity has to offer. An intoxicating blend of lights, fires, and feasts shone so much brighter for the season's short days and early darkness. Strolling around the central square of each city, we watched the crones and they, us. The native Italian old ladies dressed in black, sat and talked wildly on the edges of their town's square paused with silent smiles and scrutinized us. Together, my mother and I were a matched set in living time-lapse. (When I looked at her, my own dying affectionately looked back at me.) The sight of us walking together consistently touched people. Reactions moved across their faces, a silent inner tide invoked memories of their own dead.

IT IS A GREAT GIFT TO LIVE ENOUGH, AND LONG ENOUGH TO reconcile. This mother and daughter have always been on a journey in dramatic topography, but circumstance and strain had, at this point, loosened our tensions. My mother and I felt connected with the easy affection of sisters, but it was her new fragility that allowed it. She needed me. This was new and...I wanted to be needed by her. I found I relished walking arm in arm with her even if I didn't realize at the time how this miracle happened to be. Neediness in my family, even if mutual, was a character flaw in the framework of Betty's (and my subsequently inherited) worldview.

ANOTHER REVELATION WAS THAT ITALIANS SEEM TO HAVE A HIGH regard for old ladies—their own and the imported ones like my mother. The Italians seem to celebrate time and generations—no need to freeze time or deny death as its visage is passing the pasta each evening at the dinner table. In America, we do not love our crones. We deny them. We hide them under winched-up cosmetic surgeries, (achieved elsewhere only in skydiving free fall). In Italy, we saw appreciation everywhere. Italians loved watching them. There were even little old lady dolls.

YET ANOTHER LOVELY STRANGENESS WAS THAT, AWAY FROM THE BUS, few suspected Betty and I were Americans. Vacationing with your mother was unexpected American behavior. Why was having a beautiful, ancient woman on your arm such great camouflage from being identified as an American tourist? One Italian couple even came up and asked us for directions—in Italian. It was delicious mischief, even if only momentarily, to pretend Italian lineage. My own inner prairie woman felt exotic and my mother was very, very happy.

BY FAR THE MOST ASTOUNDING DISCOVERY WAS THAT "SANTA Claus" was a grandmother. Those dolls were of their beloved La Befana. La Befana, Italy's kind, corrugated crone, was an ancient wise woman with rosy cheeks, headscarf, big nose and—a broom.

The children write La Befana letters and post them in the chimney. La Befana brings presents for their stockings, which hang on fireplace mantels. Their presents depend on their annual behavior index: coal or sweets? The legend has it that La Befana was invited to accompany the three wise men on their journey to see the Christ child but she insisted on finishing her housework (like my own GG Sena's obsession). La Befana promised to meet up with them later. Apparently, she has been racing after them ever since with gifts and the help of her flying broom transport through windows or down chimneys.

SHE'S OBVIOUSLY WITCHY, BUT WE WERE THOUSANDS OF MILES AWAY and long past U.S. Halloween. My own rosy-cheeked crone and I pondered how a holdover from the Divine Feminine—a pre-Roman sacredness—could stay so evergreen and persistently near the hearts of Italians (and in the backyard of Vatican City). How had the Catholic seat of power tolerated La Befana after thousands of years of heavy-handed edicts, purges, and heretic corrective burnings? How was she still here?

THE REST OF LA BEFANA'S STORY TELLS THE TALE. THE CATHOLIC Church's compromise was that when each Italian holiday season ended on January 6, the La Befana dolls burn in effigy. La Befana's perennial intention is to reaffirm the bond between the family and ancestors through the annual exchange of gifts. Her bonfire sends La Befana on her journey back to the ancestors. She takes with her the negative things of the old year (pinned to her skirt), leaving behind gifts for the new of their line, and bequeathing economic prosperity for all. She stands for the continuity of family, hope, and magic at a time of year that asks us to renew ourselves or die.

La Befana comes back every year to teach Italians about loss—about releasing the old and igniting the new. Like my own dearly demented phoenix who has misplaced her matches, I needed that lesson now.

~

Phoenix Carousel

The Befana's yearly phoenix celebration has a lot to inspire a renewal by incinerating the stuff, which isn't working (and hasn't for a while). It's not like I'm going to *miss* it but even if I had a metaphysical flamethrower, there is only so much stuff that I can let go of and burn—*today*. In caregiving, we hold so much. I need the Befana *on a carousel*—to come round hourly or at least daily to release that which no longer fits who I am *now*...but to do it as I can in sweet, small steps. Incrementally works for me—chewing what I bite off.

After many villages and cities, we returned to the place we started—Milan. It was before dawn on our final day, I left my exhausted mother sleeping in the hotel while I took a walk to Milan's Duomo and the square. It was shrouded in construction scaffolding and seemed bundled up against the cold like me. With the sound of my new Italian boots echoing off buildings, I found a peaceful spot to wait on Italy's magnificent pink light. I was alone on the plaza.

The rose light arrived like fog. The sunrise held for a short pink eternity, then gave way to the astonishing pandemonium of *Italian motorcycles*. They thundered by so fast, I just caught a glimpse of a big burley La Befana astride the biggest *Ducati* painted with orange flames. That wise old woman had traded in her broom and teamed up with her consorts—the Bufanos. They were roaring cacophonous, prosperity noises. She was surrounded by handsome Italian men, honored for who she was and the wisdom of giving up what is not working. It's a good deal with lots to celebrate: being renewed, living in Italy and *playtime for our persistent phoenix of a crone.*

INSPIRE A RENEWAL—LIGHT THE MATCH. LA BEFANA'S YEARLY *Phoenix Carousel* incinerates the old, which isn't working and no longer fits who we are now.

GET EMPTY.

Let's go.

Let go.

Light the match—even if you think it's your last one.

19

CELEBRATE INCONVENIENCE

DOUBLE-DOWN WITH FUN IN THE MIDDLE OF THE MESSINESS.

Whatever the renewable balance is, I am too adaptable. I lived in the overlap of what my ex wanted or what my mother required. I did not offer them enough practice at being likewise accommodating and accepting of me. The right question, I seldom ask (and I need to) is "Am I feeling sufficiently adored?" (If only by caregiving my own self.) Why do I keep putting myself last?

I VOW TO BE MORE INCONVENIENT.

~

Celebrate Inconvenience

THIS IDEA IS AN APPETIZER TO A GREATER FEAST; IT IS A SINGLE mouthful in the feast of accepting "what is."

RIGHT NOW FROM THIS PLACE OF, PERHAPS, UNFELT AND, CERTAINLY, unripe grief, a larger celebratory buffet is inaccessible to me, but I can eat this appetizer.

IT'S ENOUGH. THIS SMALL BITE IS ABOUT *CELEBRATING THE nourishment within the inconvenience of what is.* Our first vacation was a bus tour through Italy and a lot of work for me; it was troublesome. Betty and I were problematic to the people on our tour but they rose to a level of community because they saw we *needed* them. They responded. We were difficult and it brought them together. Caregiving is inopportune, yet it unified us on the trip (and between Betty and me) in ways that being 'rugged individualists' had not (and could not).

DOUBLE-DOWN WITH FUN IN THE MIDDLE OF THE MESSINESS. (WHY is this the opposite of what most of us do?) More *doing* is not the answer. Current neuroscience agrees that those who survive stress actually *increase* their social investments (i.e. *play*) in the trenches. Integral hanging-out *between* sprints is better for the long race.

BEING INCONVENIENCED SLOWS ME DOWN. IT ALLOWS ME TO SEE another's point of view—to discern what is unchanging, and what is worth the fight to change.

ACCEPT THE SIMPLE PLEASURES OF BEING LOVED IMPERFECTLY.

CELEBRATE IT WHENEVER YOU CAN.

III

THE GARDEN OF CHANGE

20

LIVE BACKWARDS, REMEMBER BETTER

MEMORY IS A GARDEN. WHAT AND HOW I CHOOSE TO REMEMBER GROWS MY LIFE.

Celebrating inconvenience is harder than it sounds in a slow dance down the long road of caregiving. By the end, my mother had it all stripped away by her dementia—the vanity, pride, the intellect...

It didn't happen all at once. Her lapses grew thicker and deeper. A hollowness settled in—then an echoing silence. The change was gentle and transparent at first, like the scent of rain coming—close but not having yet arrived. I found myself helplessly watching the mist rise in her. During this phase of caregiving, the similarity to a certain pattern of fog repeatedly struck me—the hypnotizing siren clouds of Highway 280. Winding through the undulating grasslands of the Coast Range from the mecca of Silicon (Valley) to the innovative *Oz* of San Francisco, it uses (with no warning or apology) the San Andreas Fault line's right of way. When the-big-one-hits, its commuters will be swimming, but its famous fog's performance is *so seductive,* even fast lane venture capitalists go from all business to awestruck mesmerizing away any thought of earthquake roulette.

THIS FOG IS NOT A MIST. IT RISES THICK FROM THE PACIFIC OVER the Coast Range's hourglass hills like cream rises when whipped by an electric mixer (or shaving cream might swell in your hand from an aerosol can's pressure). When high enough, these clouds *dollop* over the lowest defense of topography and flow, filling the valley created by the fault line. All that was there a moment before is *disremembered.* Rising again, it hides the very road traveled underneath us...as we speed on and through.

MY MOTHER'S FOG, UNLIKE THESE *OBSCURING* CLOUDS, WAS *DELETING* the map upon which she traveled. She seemed to have misplaced her mightiness as dementia exposed a softness, which she had hidden in her prime. I would not, *I could not,* caregive my mother at her full strength. It was all tornados for us then. I couldn't hear anything above our thunderstorms (my own voice was in full gale).

THE PROGRESSION OF HER DECLINE DISSOLVED THE WAY OUR relationship had solidified. Our habitual critiques about excess weight turn into efforts to feed a decimated body. It was as if one was playing baseball and suddenly the rules were rugby. The mountains and valleys of one-upmanship turned into a plane of clarity where I found myself naked. I lost my trusty companion in our familiar fight. In her place was a woman without wisecrack and she was looking at me with different eyes.

Betty continued re-experiencing people; she lived by repurposing those who showed up. She imagined her caregivers as long-lost companions or she helped herself to recasting my friends who came to visit. Her days were *full* of social events.

INSTEAD OF REMEMBERING MY MOTHER SCARED WHEN SHE WAS dying, or that I might have contributed to her demise by allowing all those prescription pills, or any number of dark mother stories of my upbringing, I see us sitting in our sunny San Francisco apartment—in a sweet spot of time. We are soaking up the laid-back San Francisco sun in a corner window, looking at the western skyline: Pacific Ocean and Presidio Forest. We are rocking on a peaceful edge of our lives. We are not broken. In our dailyness, we are whole, and happy in the sweet small steps we were able to take together. I remember those moments and feel pretty great.

Live Backwards. ***Remember Better.***

THIS IS MY SEASON, TOO. THIS IS MY TIME.

I want to choose well how I spend the rest of it, and be deeply satisfied with my choices. Dwelling on the "what ifs" and regrets of the past are a pity party. What we did or never did (or was done to us) is over unless we keep it alive by picking at the scabs. Remembering better is something quite different. It is not judgment but discernment with adult eyes. It is a mainstay rule of caregiving and the endgame to a good life. We are going forward together now on an inter-dependent journey; I need you to help me see better and you need me for similar reasons.

MEMORY IS A GARDEN. WHAT AND HOW I CHOOSE TO REMEMBER *grows my life.*

MOST OF MY RULES ARE ABOUT STAYING ALIVE FOR THE MARATHON (or endless sprints) of caregiving: *Diva Breathe, Stay Full, Play Daily,* and *Stop. Rest.* Repeat the first eight and start again. Those rules keep you alive; the first eight keep you in shape. Being happy at it is another thing entirely. In response to the question, *What is the secret to happiness as you age?* The lively, lovely 108 year old replied:

> "Instead of forward, I am living backwards…I look where it is good. I know about the bad. There has to be the bad, but I look at the good thing."
>
> — ALICE HERZ-SOMMER AT 108 YEARS OLD, A PIANIST, A HOLOCAUST SURVIVOR 1903—2014

Alice Hertz-Sommer was an optimist. With her focus on the good things, she outlived her twin sister, the pessimist, by several decades. Letting anxiety and fear rule you, reduces your life by decades. Looking to 'where it is good' extends your life both in quantity and *quality.*

WHAT MAKES ME REMEMBER CRITICISM TWENTY TIMES LOUDER than a compliment?

Habits are laid down chemically in our brains. Neurons fire and impulses travel on well-worn thought trails throughout my synapses. These thoughts ruts seek out our well-traveled mental roads—*literally.*

CAN I JUST *CHOOSE* A BETTER, HAPPIER MOMENT ON WHICH to focus?

Or simply remember differently? I get so caught up in the fear, criticism and anxiety, could it be that simple—to stop running in my own little hamster wheel? Shifting to some *more interesting* story—or something more *worth* doing?

> "The only true voyage of discovery, the *only fountain of Eternal Youth,* would be not to visit strange lands but to possess other eyes, to behold the universe through the eyes of another, of a hundred others, to behold the hundred universes that each of them beholds, that each of them is.
>
> — MARCEL PROUST, THE CAPTIVE 1871-1922

Do we dare to re-remember? To retell and rewrite? What if we just woke up and translated the old stories into a different language in which we understand that *all people* act to their level of skill. They do the best they can in the moment—with what they have. Why not reinterpret my stories in the light of my current more-adult understandings? Then my history changes. It sets me up to cascade forward. Who I am changes. I am free. There is nothing to forgive.

FORGIVE ANYWAY. THIS IS THE GOAL OF A BETTER REMEMBERING. We don't have to get dementia to do this. (I believe it may be the best way not to *get* dementia.) There is freedom here. Live backwards. Remember better.

21

MOBIUS REGRETS

CONGRATULATE YOURSELF. REGRETS CAN BE AN INFINITE LOOP TO BETTER.

As confusing as *Live Backwards, Remember Better* is, I believe it to be worth considering. Little else has moved me forward as quickly as seeing my stuckness from another perspective. However, to activate this superpower, I must be more willing than willful—which is not one of my natural gifts, nor was it Betty's.

HER LIFE ALL WENT SMOOTHLY FOR A TIME, TOO, UNTIL IT STARTED looping. She just worked harder at doing the same thing—with *different* people. Betty did not change but she changed husbands. Later, she tried repurposing people—allowing the same beings (such as me) to switch slots (daughter became buddy; daughter became mother). Betty kept repeating the pattern, trying again to *force* it to work, as is the way of prairie grit. She was sure that the next streetcar (i.e. jobs, husbands, tax seasons) would be *the one.* Then she would be happy. She focused on the pursuit of *happy* and not the actual satisfaction of ever *just being* it. She never altered, until dementia did it for her.

Tempered in the fires of her experience, her prairie grit melted like sand does into glass, she metamorphosed (and in some ways metastasized) into the sparkling but fundamentally fragile glass figurine of the mother with whom I grew to adulthood. When she did break, almost sixty years later, she shattered.

Ours was an enthrallment, of sorts. Her narrative would not let her adjust; mine would not let me quit.

Mobius Regrets

What is a regret? I know *better* now, how and what *not* to do.

I have changed and *learned* something. Congratulate yourself. You are wiser. That's progress—it's not shameful. My mother never had regrets to my knowledge. To have regrets means you must change.

Life seems to be a cosmic crapshoot. Screwing up is part of it. It's messy.

Regrets are mile markers on the road. Our personalized path through life (as it seems *made* for us to learn what we need) can get *a little twisted.* This is a good thing. With only one twist, the circular loop of ribbon, which previously had both an inner and an outer side, becomes an infinite loop where there is only one side—and one path. With that single half turn, you now have a Mobius. It's the worldwide symbol for recycling.

CONGRATULATE YOURSELF. REGRETS CAN BE AN INFINITE LOOP TO *better.*

WHEN WE CAN GET TO THIS...THIS LOOP OF WHOLENESS (I.E. nothing's broken...it is what it is), then there is nothing to forgive because it is all part of it. Every piece, every prayer is part of the journey. All the rules that I have earned, learned and offered to you, lead up to this ripeness. My attitude is accepting and open to using it all—but reinterpreted and repurposed.

WITH A FEW OF THESE MATURING ROTATIONS, I STARTED TO BE aware that I landed in the same place—the spot *in which I did not want to be.* Before you bootstrap yourself back up into the same self-denying downward cycle (that must again, by definition, land you on your knees in that same puddle), regret it, and resolve to choose better. We choose from the best at hand—love or fear. What do you want?

WE CANNOT ALWAYS BE RIGHT; REGRETS ARE PART OF IT BUT WE don't want to get stuck moping in the hallway before the next door opens. Dwelling is useless. Fixating on tough times is worse.

> "Regret for lost time, is more lost time."
>
> — MASON COOLEY

WE CAN LEARN FROM REGRET AND RECYCLE IT.

But, hey—if you're not there, don't twist yourself into a pretzel.

Stop. Rest. You're normal and this is the part of the road where we have lots of company. Wait *Here*—or go grab a friend for a good *Cackle* over cocktails. Do some quiet quantum composting (or trash talking). Get it off your chest and let it go. Prepare your ground for some new seeds. Nourish yourself—go eat something happy: *Mangia, Mangia.*

Start again tomorrow. It is like a shower, we need to practice daily.

22

IMPROV "WHAT IS"

UNDERNEATH ALL THE CHAOS OF "WHAT IS", LOVE WAITS TO PLAY.

Whether a circular and celebratory *Mobius Regrets* or one long, linear unexamined life, you're gonna *Keep Moving* through. The door to the next thing will open on its own. If I come into this world, I will have to go out.

EVERYONE DOES IT—EVEN THE FUNNY AND THE FAMOUS.

> "I do not fear death. I had been dead for billions and billions of years before I was born, and had not suffered the slightest inconvenience from it."
>
> — MARK TWAIN

> "Now he has departed from this strange world a little ahead of me. That means nothing. People like us, who believe in physics, know that the distinction between past, present, and future is only a stubbornly persistent illusion."

—ALBERT EINSTEIN, UPON LEARNING OF THE DEATH OF A LIFELONG FRIEND, IN A MARCH 1955 LETTER.

The Goodbye Theatre

As I have been in this 'strange world' a while, it is easy to see how we, in the US of A, are black belts in death aversion. A little more of our 'persistent illusion' can make a difference, at the end—enough to say goodbye or find those serendipitous opportunities for reconciliation, reconnection, or forgiveness. Hospice can offer a comfortable space for sweetness to happen before we touch down to the final mystery. When deaf, dumb, and blind as to how our own folks did their dying, the photo finish to a good death will be more of a crapshoot. No one has yet avoided it... with or without practice (and with or without good pain meds).

Some families do well-meaning torture on their beloveds in hopeless and painful procedures because *we are ourselves* afraid of change—and that ultimate change. Most people wait too long to move into *comfortable* ending days (which are possible). Then, they are caught in a panic of *no-time-left.*

Mindful caregiving is about serving and companioning in a respectful peer relationship. As Rachel Naomi Remen offers, it is very different than helping or fixing as a mental framework (the helper/fixer role has a power dynamic placing us above the patient.[4]). I have noticed that on the frontlines of love, families are all of these but in the end—for a good death—there is only one path: serving where we are equal. You can easily feel the difference ('You poor thing..." vs. 'Here are some options, what works for you, today?') Loss complicates our ability to see clearly. A good death respectfully allows *the patient* to steer.

As caregivers, we must ask, and re-ask the question, "What do you want?" or "What would *they* want, if they were still able to tell us?" It takes time until families are able to let go enough to answer. I get it (and I did it, too)—not the torture part but the paralysis of *coming* losses. It's impossible to be fully ready for such a loss; it is possible to *Be Willing.* I have seen death be a great gift for (and to all) present—when we are willing.

Improv 'What is'

Architects fix their designs from the fluid sketches on their drawing boards. After construction, they make final plans of what was *actually* built. An 'as built' plan documents 'What is'. From this moment on, only human maintenance will resist the forces of nature to keep the building standing.

Landscape architects do the same but have few illusions that growing things, which are much of the primary components of our designs, will stay the *same.* A garden changes *what is* in every moment with growth, seasons, death, and (unskillful) weed whackers.

Staying the same, for a garden, means *it's dead.*

Human beings design with life, too—we co-create. We can't help it.

We do our best to imagine and prepare for what will be tomorrow or in twenty years, but things change as constantly as the tax code. It is natural and normal for "What is" to quickly turn into "Shit happens." It's up to those people still standing to improvise a way to grow and bloom anyway.

Starting each moment as a blank slate is the domain of improvisational theatre.

Fixating on *no change is* the architecture of death. Saying "Yes…and", allowing things to open up (and connect) is the garden of improv. If we say 'No" to dementia's reality, we stop the flow, and the *renewing* relationship between us. Say "Yes and…" for opportunities to grow. Many families reasonably resist dementia's reality with Alzheimer's orientation boards, standard memory therapy, photos of family with name labels, because to lose shared memories is to deny who we belong to, who we *are*. We resist going into their world to be *with them* and insist that they come into ours which they no longer share. It's like speaking Chinese to Spaniards and expecting them to answer in English. (Seems a little *demented*?)

> "The only man I know who behaves sensibly is my tailor; he takes my measurements anew each time he sees me. The rest go on with their old measurements and expect me to fit them."

— GEORGE BERNARD SHAW, MAN AND SUPERMAN.

UNDERNEATH ALL THE CHAOS OF "WHAT IS", LOVE WAITS TO PLAY.

NINE YEARS INTO CAREGIVING, WITH TWO TO GO, I TRIED something new with my mother. A friend asked, "Why not change your history to something Betty always wanted?" She suggested, "Since your mother won't remember anyway, tell her something joyful about the people *she misses*. Make it real, whether it's true or not."

YOU WANT ME TO *LIE* TO HER?" I WAS RESPECTFULLY SHOCKED. I was, even then, still taking caregiving *very seriously*. How could I play around with illness or joke with our *memories*? I then thought again. She no longer *shared* much of our history.

I RECONSIDERED WHAT I KNEW TO BE GOOD AND TRUE.

A REGRET OF MY MOTHER'S WILLINGLY (AND JOYFULLY) OFFERED itself to me. My mother didn't have many regrets but Betty always wished she had taken her mother, Annie, to Denmark. Copenhagen was my Great-Grandmother Sena's hometown. The next time Betty asked me why her mother, Annie, "did not visit her (and why was she angry with me)?" I was ready. (I knew, of course, that being dead for twenty-five years was not an acceptable excuse.) So, I *made stuff up*...which is improv[5]. For realism, I included my grandmother's sidekick, Alpha in the story.

"Yes and...they aren't here; they're traveling, honey. Alpha and Annie got a great deal on first class tickets last week. They flew off to Copenhagen to see the old country—Denmark."

Betty absolutely lit up. (It was a silent *Cackle*.)

Feeling a bit more confident, because she was so happy, I elaborated. "Yes and...I think their itinerary puts them in Odense right now, visiting Hans Christian Andersen's and Grandmother Sena's girlhood town."

"That *is* so wonderful." Betty looked straight at me, awake and amazed. "I always wanted to take her and she finally got to go... *Perfect*." In that moment, she was joyfully participating in a *new* and better tale.

I looked at her. She was *so happy*. I saw this moment from a distance, knowing that I would be receiving joy from it for the rest of my lifetime.

Then I added, "Yes and...we should be getting a postcard from them very soon."

23

MAGIC METTLE

TRY THESE MAGIC WORDS: "WHAT YOU ARE IS ALREADY AWESOME.' WELCOME HOME.

Betty improvised motherhood like I did caregiving. Seeing no reasonable middle path to being both a mother and a businesswoman, she did both anyway. My bio-father was long gone but my adopted dad, John W. Hager, was a steady, loving presence. Even with his help, *Improv What Is* became an essential survival skill of motherhood for Betty. She delegated a great deal of it...to competent and loving surrogates.

Mother Manna

As the first generation of American women to have a choice —to have suffrage—she explored her options. She knew how untrustworthy the world could be for a smart, ambitious woman. It was post-WWII and the set of *Mad Men* was her reality show.

She gave me her very best lessons. I know this. At the same time, she was not attending and seeing me as much as mirroring back the great need to *fix my flaws* as a matter of *my own survival.* I marinated in that idea, and let it get baked into me—long before I knew I was cooking. The point, now, is that I am still, and always have been, *the cook.*

ACCEPTING AND APPRECIATING YOUR KID FOR WHO THEY ARE, (BUT staying well short of helicopter mothering) is the billion year-old home recipe for making resilient adults. They have a better chance to bounce confidently in an uncertain world. Betty had a good mother, Annie, who believed in her. I had Annie's belief, too, *but I didn't believe her.* Perhaps Betty didn't believe her either, when she was a youngster. Neither of us took the approval *into* ourselves. Betty wanted the approval of her first string, her father, and I wanted her's.

IN THE END, IT'S REALLY NONE OF MY BUSINESS—THE WHY OR THE how come. We get what we get. Blame is wasted effort...from the vantage point of a good life, but forgiveness is essential. My sight is so limited into why my (or anyone's) significant and beloved others do what they do, if they *Do* (not) *Bother* to speak their truth into clarity. Perhaps they never looked up from the chase of something (*anything*) better.

WE GET WHAT WE GET AND MAKE THE REST OF IT UP. OR, PERHAPS I came into this world with buckets of leftover garbage ideas to work through and (quantum) compost. From the perspective of a good life and a good end, it doesn't matter the origin of the manure—just the efficacy of my personal compost pile.

I AM NOT SO MUCH BRIMMING WITH RESENTMENTS AT THIS POINT,

as looking for executables. I need to *poof-be-gone* what I suspect was my mother's judgment early on (and now my subcutaneous geology) at not finding her daughter all that interesting. This (subconscious) substrata is, however, so inaccessible at this point that a magic wand would be useful (which I seem to have misplaced). Restoration and renewal is about growing deeper, more sustaining roots—*of my own making*. Perhaps a magic *trowel of remembering better* for all the good mothers who *have* loved me? Or manna from heaven would work, too.

HOW CAN I FRACK THIS WATER FROM A STONE—THAT I AM *WORTHY and well made*? It's like brain surgery with a shovel—tricky business.

> "Death and life is in the power of the tongue."
>
> — PROVERBS 18:21

EVEN IF YOU HAVE BEEN ON THE PLANET A WHILE, IF YOU DIDN'T GET enough good word-food or healthy mirroring as a kid, you have issues. Ask a shrink (or one of your exes). Malnutrition is in my marrow and *I-am-sick-of-it*. If you are pooh-poohing the notion, as my bootstrapped self did for years, this metaphysical vitamin deficiency will just get hungrier until you attend.

IT'S A CONFIDENCE IN MYSELF THAT ARISES AS (AND WITH) MY CORE Earth. My missing ingredient (for a good life) looked like confidence in the world but I misread the recipe for years. It was, instead, acceptance and appreciation *in my inner world.*

Caregiving's exhaustion stressed me to the point that my survival *necessitated* a better way. I reassessed the being in the mirror *deciding* to value my *aptitudes*—my seed gifts—*as enough.* I replanted myself within the humus of *providential resources,* to find that I had more than enough to grow *my life.*

The grace of rain did (and does) the rest.

We water the seeds of what we want to grow *with our intention.* We are the gardeners who cultivate the best seedings in ourselves and in others. It's a very human superpower that looks like *magic.* It is the mirroring of unconditional positive regard[7] for yourself and others. It is what I do daily at bedside.

I am planting seeds that will grow what I need, even if I must *Wait Here,* before I see any sprouts. It's about the renewable inner means to grow—well and *enough.* I have enough and have what I need for what is mine to do.

How can I inject this belief of 'enoughness' straight into my veins?

Can I own, at this point, the deep knowing that everything will be okay—even though I don't see how? If so, I can let whatever outcomes or feedback from the world land where they will—boom or bust. Like a tree in a metaphysical October, I am *aware that winter is coming but I am blazing in brilliant colors* anyway—allowing my leaves to fall, wherever they will because I have roots...*and a full aquifer.*

Magic Mettle

MAGIC HAPPENED. LIKE DOROTHY, WE FOUND *HOME* IN NAVIGATING the potholes on the road.

It seems we had to (I had to...) *do* the Yellow Brick journey, to be ripe *enough* (or empty enough...) for the (impossibly) simple insight of Glinda's instructions in perennial wisdom.

MY ANTIDOTE TO THE FEAR OF *NOT ENOUGH* HAS BEEN HERE ALL along. By sitting still and listening, Glinda the Good Witch has apparated within the largesse of grief just in time. The epiphany of the ruby slippers lies in the arms of my (inner) good mother as I scoop up the fearful pieces of me...*and hold them.* Use whatever name, or face that comforts you, but these super powers are femme—manna-making-mettle.

ANNIE KNEW THIS.

TRY THESE MAGIC WORDS: "WHAT YOU ARE *IS ALREADY AWESOME —just right.*"

YOU ARE HOME. YOU BELONG. WE WANT YOU HERE."

> "Are you ready now? Close your eyes and just tap your heels together *three* times and think to yourself: there is no place like home...there is no place like home...there is no place like home."

— GLINDA EXPLAINING TO DOROTHY HOW TO GO BACK HOME. MGM'S THE WIZARD OF OZ, 1939, BY L. FRANK BAUM

Remember that you have the power (and you have had it all along).

I QUIET THE CHORUS OF THE 'NOT ENOUGH'S' ON THE OCCASIONS that parts of me get triggered and don't feel safe. It happens all the time, when you risk. It *especially* happens when I try and play it safe.

> "Rubbish. Be gone! You have *no* power here. Be gone before someone drops a house on you, too."
>
> — GLINDA PROTECTING DOROTHY FROM THE WRATH OF THE WICKED WITCH IN MGM'S THE WIZARD OF OZ 1939, BY L. FRANK BAUM

This knowing is so deep it's almost instinct...but it may be *learned.*

IT'S A CONFIDENCE, WHICH UNDERPINS THE ABILITY TO HAVE FAITH— when we don't know. (Multiplied by millions, a healthy economy depends on it.) It is what gives us creative powers to prosper in the busts *and* the booms of caregiving and renewing community.

MOTHERS DIE BUT GOOD SELF-NURTURING NEVER STOPS WHILE WE ourselves are alive. For all our collective inner-child(s) left behind and longing (for something succulent...), we can be our *own* good mothers. This more loving inner voice speaks to me in nature, in religious iconography, in poetry, in prayer and in the very potholes of our constitutional pursuit of happiness. It is not selfish, but a hotline to the Holy One of Many Names in the Kingdom of God within—as we understand it to be.

We need you here. Say it now, 'What I am is already awesome.'

See if things don't start aligning for you. What have you got to lose but the wicked, self-defeating voices? Your mother-mirror is healing gold. It's alchemy that makes life *just work out.*

24

GOT BLESSING?

VALIDATION IS FOR PARKING—BUT HAVING A BLESSING IS A CONSTANTLY REFILLING GAS TANK.

My lack of feeling a fitness for this world was something a *good mother* could have given with some *Magic Mettle.* If Betty had been a more lavishly attentive mother, would I have been as doggedly devoted a daughter? Such an enduring caregiver? Or even who I am now?

ON THE OTHER HAND, HOW COULD SHE GIVE ME SOMETHING THAT she never had? We both required what our heroes withheld—a blessing. It's a bestowing of a fundamental rightness that permeates through all our calcifications and constructed protections. It has the power to transform—everything.

Got Blessing?

DID YOUR PARENTS GIVE YOU THEIR BLESSING OR TEACH YOU TO *earn* love?

MUST YOU PROVE YOURSELF? ARE YOU SEEKING APPROVAL IN THE world, or from the opinions of others? Love was my carrot cantilevered just out of the reach of a yoked-up donkey luring me to *Keep Moving*—either for my own good or for that of someone else.

VALIDATION *IS FOR PARKING*—BUT HAVING A BLESSING IS A constantly refilling gas tank.

ON THE SURFACE, THIS RULE SOUNDS CLICHÉD (AND PERHAPS banal...), but surprisingly it is another superpower for a good life. It is the difference between a cup that 'runneth over' versus one with holes poked in it, which constantly leaks our enough-ness.

A BLESSING IS BESTOWED. IT IS A GIFT. BEING PURCHASED MAKES IT untrustworthy. It loses its power, as it does when we earn it. Only if it is given freely, does it have the power to *amend us.*

IT OFFERS BALANCE IN THE WORLD WHEN PLANS FAIL AND STORIES end.

A BLESSING IS A SOFTER LANDING PLACE. IT IS A SEED OF *CERTAINTY* planted within. It is simple well-being in our inevitable human valleys, and the superpower of knowing beyond appearance that you are okay and, perhaps, that *it will all be* okay, even if you don't know how.

THE UNIVERSE *WANTS ME HERE.*

WHERE DO I, AS THE FRACTAL PROGENY OF MY OH-SO-HUMAN parents get a blessing? Some lucky kids, as with *Magic Mettle,* had parents who paid real attention—but not *too much* attention. Those parents who fed their approval to their kids—believing in their offspring and telling them so.

BETTY AND I BOTH SPENT A LIFETIME OF TRYING TO EXECUTE success goals given to us by our heroes—so we might earn a blessing: mine from her—and her's from her father. Then we would be *enough.* Her father died abruptly. I don't believe she ever got a blessing from him—but I gave her mine. Betty gave me her's after a long life and dying process but, at that point, I didn't need it. *I had made my own.*

IT'S A LOT TO ASK.

Effective parents find the complicated, dynamic, good-life balance between their own lives, well lived, and their children's. It's everything to tending and growing a garden. Even as a child I have a part. I become a *chosen one* when I take the blessing *in*—receiving and accepting it. Especially as an adult, when it is my turn to till the good earth under my feet—then I become the gardener of my own good life.

I STUBBORNLY WANTED FROM BETTY WHAT SHE COULD NOT GIVE. AS a child, there were others around who blessed me but I discounted them. The father of my heart, John W., was standing watch. My grandmother, Annie, had her heart open for me, and many others since that time—Albertina was one.

No more do I discount their gifts. I see them and bless them back.

Even if you weren't originally a chosen one, if we are still breathing, we can give the gift of blessing...ourselves—to ourselves. The skill sets to address monsters under our beds are learned. I give you mine now: knowing you are enough, may you feel the good food in your veins, so to use all the gifts that you have been given.

You can upgrade yourself with a blessing. (Hint; you *are* the blessing.)

25

WILD WITHIN

NOW IS THE TIME FOR WILDNESS, TEMPERANCE....AND LAUGHTER—DREAMING A LITTLE WILDER AND WIDER.

In post-caregiving exhaustion and grief, I lost my way. I needed directions—something subtle like flashing lights on an airport runway would have done nicely. A self-igniting torch would also have worked...to light the way. Coincidently, the Greek maiden goddess, Artemis, has shown up in my life. She has one, as well as a wicked bow and quiver. (I yearn to be *that* well accessorized.)

I HAVE BEGUN RUMMAGING AROUND IN MY HISTORY AND FAMILY narratives to find my way. As a kid who loved wildness, it occurs to me, this goddess would have been good to know when growing up. She was a fearless protector of undomesticated wild things, girls, pregnant and childbearing women, and children who couldn't protect themselves. In myth, she, as a virgin goddess, hung out with a bunch of carefree nymphs who danced ecstatically around in the woods with live baskets of plants on their heads, making like happy, thriving, growing things. (It's not so hard to be carefree when you have the original archer goddess watching over you...)

GRANDMOTHERLY WILDNESS

Betty's wildness was more Dionysian only after the doors of commerce had closed for the day. She drank and generally appreciated imbibing, unlike her paternal grandmother, Zip (short for Zilpha), who was dedicated to temperance and prohibition. That never stopped Betty from regularly invoking her paternal Scottish grandmother by insisting that we drink up...(and not waste anything) "because Zip is sitting on your shoulder..." (Conveniently omitting her tee-totaling pledge of the times to *never* touch the stuff, when finishing the last round.)

GLIMPSES INTO MY GRANDMOTHER ANNIE'S YOUTHFUL ENERGY were anything but staunch puritanism. It was more the Scandinavian way—to live and let live (invoking her own Danish mother, Sena). Annie did not share her mother-in-law's staunch views. She was only thirty-one when prohibition ended in 1933.

ON OCCASION, BETTY GOT HER MOTHER TO LOOSEN UP WITH A sweet cocktail of some kind. (Annie favored drinks with little umbrellas or cream sherry.) Betty's drink was always a manly scotch-on-the-rocks "with a twist". I looked for opportunities to tease my grandmother about her drinking, which she rarely did. Or I might make up something about how she 'passed out.' She play-scolded me back, and pointed or pinched me into squealing laughter.

"YOU CAN GO THERE FOR LYING, THE SAME AS YOU CAN FOR

stealing," was her standard response which was usually accompanied by a wagging finger.

I INFERRED STORIES OF THE YOUNGER ANNIE FROM HER occasionally cheeky sense of humor. Here are a couple of ditties as evidence. It's a limerick recited by Betty and Annie (when she did imbibe).

> *I never drink martinis*
> *One or two at the most,*
> *Three I'm under the table,*
> *Four I'm under my host.*

MY SOFT, SWEET-SMELLING, AND CREPEY-SKINNED GRANDMOTHER would smile and sparkle with a moment of wildness. For a moment, I could see her foxtrotting with her hunky, young Fred under the stars to the tunes on the local Depression-era radio broadcast from Cain's Ballroom. They danced, (even if they couldn't afford the ten-cent admission price to Tulsa's nouveau riche nightspot). She then resumed her dignified, earthy, and loving presence. It was all very deniable and innocent but it was a clue. She had not forgotten her young self to which we, her progeny, would never truly be privy.

THERE WAS A SECOND LIMERICK IN MY FEMME LINEAGE THAT ANNIE recited. After she passed, Betty and I took on the tradition by making it a spontaneous duet of honor.

"Here's to the girl with the little red shoes," Betty usually started and paused here for me with open palms—cueing me to continue.

"She liked her whisky, she liked her booze." I could not help, at this point, but smile.

"She lost her cherry, but that's no sin."

The last line was usually in unison." "She still had the box that the cherry came in. "

No matter what hideous finality was on our plate, happiness happened in us when we recited this. A strange, small window opened in which an inner too-loud-to-be-lady-like cackle might be transmitted backwards in time, so Annie could hear. It was membership in the sisterhood-of-whatever-works.

Even in her ending days—these limericks delighted unsuspecting visitors to "our" hospice home away from home to chuckle amid their own catastrophic losses. It *was* funny but it was also an important moment *to be seen* as more than one-more-old-lady-and-her-middle-aged-daughter. We claimed a moment of our identity back and we watered our roots, remembering our long-dead Annie and her once mischievous *goodness*. It was a time-traveling moment shared, and then we popped back into the mundane—just another old lady and her daughter—but we were *laughing.*

Wild Within

NOW IS THE TIME FOR WILDNESS, TEMPERANCE...*AND LAUGHTER.*

NO MATTER HOW MANY THOUSANDS OF YEARS WE HAVE BEEN OUT OF balance between our masculine reason and our feminine intuition, the pristine, unadulterated forest ecosystem is available to begin the balance *again if we remember.* (Now is the only time it was ever available, if you want to get nit picky about the metaphysics.) The path between 'What is...and what I want', is available within—in the wildest (and widest) of possibilities.

WHAT MAKES ME COME ALIVE? THAT IS THE RIGHT QUESTION.

I HAVE NOT DARED TO DREAM LIKE A KID DREAMS FOR A LONG, LONG time. What are my wildest dreams? I am sorry to acknowledge that I have reduced, edited, and confabulated them to the likely and the probable for so long, it is hard to imagine them in their primal largess.

MY TIME IS LIMITED HERE ON THE PLANET. I SEE THIS EMBODIED reality every day as a hospice chaplain (and in the mirror). What I choose to do is a *valuable currency*—perhaps the ultimate, universal denomination—the worth of a life. What do I want? What is mine to do? These are terrifying (and wonderful) questions.

What would happen if I didn't limit my dream from the outset? Perhaps more possibilities for my post-caregiving life? Right now, in grief, I am too confused to embrace the *entire* wild world of possibilities but I am not stuck. I am taking sweet small steps in the wilderness. Reasonably oriented is all I have right now...but it's enough.

Channeling my inner Artemis, I am willing to dream a little *wilder* and wider.

My mother had bigger dreams and more Artemis in her than I. She played hard. She dared to *love* the hunt—and the kill.

Get lost in what inspires you. I found myself there.

26

RIGHT WEEDING

WHAT'S THE DIFFERENCE BETWEEN A WEED AND A FLOWER? IT'S A LOT LIKE REAL ESTATE.

Being a caregiver is humbling. So is gardening. Wildness, weeds and "what is" fight with what I have planned. We've got the noisy bird chatter of cants in our heads eating up our initiatives; sometimes we have only shallow soil to work with where my less endowed root system is challenged. Then there is thorny anxiety and fear to choke out sunlight, and starve us in the dark[8]. Our families plant in us the best seeds they know—family-tested and trusted. (No matter how wrong or inappropriate that turns out to be.)

Right Weeding

OPTIMUM GROWING CONDITIONS DON'T MATTER.

Finding the balance between welcoming surprises and protecting the seeds, I have planted can be a lot of work. Finding my right-fitting crop of joy is what matters.

THERE ARE MYSTERIOUS FORCES INVOLVED HERE.

How many wonderful things that happened to me, were not in my plans? Many…so, so many. (Who am I kidding?) *Most.*

AT SOME POINT, WE TAKE OVER OUR OWN CULTIVATION. Complaining about the prior management is useless.

WE FORGIVE SO NEW BARE GROUND CLEARS AND SHOWS ITSELF TO US for planting. We learn better—more regenerative, wiser wisdoms —or we continue to loop, unaware, with the old ones until our crops die (or we do). As the gardener of my life, I am facilitating, nurturing, keeping watch, adapting, *and* maintaining curiosity about the unknown (i.e., good-mothering or self-cultivation), but I am also weeding. I am clear there are some things that no longer *serve* me.

WHAT'S THE DIFFERENCE BETWEEN A WEED AND A FLOWER? IT'S A lot like real estate.

LOCATION, LOCATION, LOCATION. DOES IT FIT THE LOCALE AND THE situation?

IT'S ABOUT A *RIGHT* FIT.

They could be the same plant—but in one human landscape it's a weed, and in the other an award-winning flower. Pampas grass is adapted in its native Africa, but in Northern California where it has naturalized, it commonly hurts animals that are not adapted to eating small spiny thorns on its leaves. We don't see a 'weed' as useful because it does not serve us or belong. (My weeds are of 'not enough' and they have an unfortunately robust taproot.) These are *weeds* in my good life—so are fear and anxiety.

My postmortem (post-Betty) life is not the 'garden' that I planned to tend.

My plot was rototilled by death. It wasn't until the protective over-story of my elders fell that I felt the full exposure of the world. The thing about gardening with *'What Is,'* is that it is not clear until you try a few times, growing a crop, or a relationship, or a business, if it will bear fruit—or if it even *belongs* to me. Perhaps it's an imposter's Cuckoo-egg of a story in *my* garden.

> "Everybody is a genius. But if you judge a fish by its ability to climb a ladder, it will live its whole life believing that it is stupid."
>
> — ALBERT EINSTEIN

My life stopped working. I got stuck. Grief made me see differently.

Perhaps I will plant something more fitting while I'm here in the muck of loss…or should I try again to do the same story over but *better this time?* I need to *Wait Here* and feel what needs to be felt—for me right now: the hurt, sadness, disappointment...and the satisfaction and joy. Then I will know what to weed or feed.

Make a garden from what you already have—it's enough.

WATCH FOR THE SEEDLINGS THAT WILL GROW A BETTER LIFE FOR you. Water the happy and delightful; weed the rest. Like those seeds in the dark, we are waiting for the conditions to spark life again.

27

JOYOUS WAGER

AN INHERENT BELIEF IN THE GOODNESS OF THE UNSEEN IS A BET WORTH PLACING.

In the almost six years since my mother's death, I have weeded some of my basic assumptions. I have been transported and altered by upside-down unknowables.

REMEMBERING BACK, I KNEW IMMEDIATELY AFTER MY MOTHER'S death that I was as bad at grief as she was. Impatient for the pain to be over, *Stop Rest* was not in my skill set. *Diva Breathe* was about all I could muster. I was driving fast with a happy face sticky-note over my gas gauge.

GRATEFULLY, MY GRIEF COUNSELOR'S BARITONE WAS WITH ME AND slowing me down.

"MY LIFE SHOULD BE GROWING BACK BY NOW...BUT I FEEL SO —*empty*." I had satisfaction from the decade of care I gave my mother but I was more astounded than gratified. I had somehow managed it...but now I was in a dark place. When I tried to find words to explain this further to my counselor, I saw only bare, black earth...*steaming.*

I TRIED AGAIN, "I FEEL LIKE COMPOST THAT'S TOO HOT TO BE USEFUL —I'm still *cooking.*"

HIS EYEBROWS ROSE. *"HMMM..."* HE LOOKED MORE PERPLEXED... (and clearly *was not* a gardener).

"LOOK, IT'S ALL TOO MUCH." I SAID, "IT IS ALL TOO F--KING MUCH to *digest...*"

HE GOT THAT AND LOOKED AT ME WITH KINDNESS. *DID HE JUST SHIFT in his seat to shield a shudder?* I never swear; my good girl won't let me but my good woman allows it sometimes for rare emphasis. *(Neither of these good 'selves' are very lively but they are loyal.)*

I WAS TRANSPORTED BACK TO MY MOTHER'S ENDING DAYS IN HER hospice bed. She, too, was stuck on replay—in a loop of longing.

"I DIDN'T DO ENOUGH," SHE SAID, MURMURING THE VOICES IN MY own head (she put them there) that if we just did a bit more...we could make all of it go right. Here I was again reaching deeper, leaning into her ear, at bedside, and reminding her of how much she *did* do. (I adored soothing her with these whispered love notes.)

AGAIN, I SAID TO HER (AND TO MY GRIEF COUNSELOR A FEW MONTHS later), "I am feeling lighter these days. I am not afraid of other people's judgments. I am so much kinder to myself and some good things are moving the business along, too."

IN MY HEAD I HEARD HER SAY, "GOOD". HER VOLUPTUOUS 'OLD SELF' rose in that moment, coming back within her emaciated frame. Betty continued, "I don't want you to be afraid. I am proud of you; never forget that."

"I WON'T." I AM GOING TO KEEP THAT PURRED PROMISE. (IT'S TIME to stick those endearing notes on my own forehead.)

A Joyous Wager

EVERY CHOICE I MAKE IS AN INVESTMENT IN ONE THING...AND (sadly) *not* another.

CAREGIVING IS A BEAUTIFUL EXAMPLE OF THIS. IT IS A COMMITMENT —even a covenant. It takes time and resources away from something else that I could be doing. I willingly chose to do it, (and would again) but I am aware of time now as a bank account. Caregiving and death have changed my perception of time. As a hospice chaplain, I know (and have seen) the sources of unlimited love, light and mercy at bedside, but have no notions that my time here will be unlimited. Like everyone else, I came into this world and I will go out.

Am I scared to move on because my best might be over? My best people gone? My best day lived? Of course, it's my same old 'not enough'—habit energy. My focus on fear will plant more seeds of fear (and grow those weeds). These are *worry* questions and already have implied negative answers.

The truth is I don't know—and *'don't know'* is neutral.

Neutral is centered—and full of *possibilities*. What stops me from being *curious* about them? Quantum scientists only understand about four percent of the universe. The rest is 'dark'—dark matter, dark energy, as yet unknown and unseen. That is a lot of space for some new options.

> "Never put a period, where God has put a comma."
>
> — GRACIE ALLEN, AMERICAN COMIC, 1895-1964

Life can be risky (and punctuation matters).

It's about having solid ground (*Got Blessing?*) to trust that I still have enough when things change. It's about faith that the universe is a friendly place and *wants me here*. From this secure ground, a place of enoughness, my focus can be on dancing with the questions.

Loss is a bitch until you realize, the cranky old broad is a great friend. La Befana and her broom cleans house with forgiveness and renewal. Let go of what is not working. Bet on Einstein's friendly universe.

> "Faith is a free surrender and a joyous wager on the unseen, unknown, untested goodness of God."
>
> — MARTIN LUTHER

WILLINGNESS TO RISK ALLOWS US TO VENTURE OUT AND GROW things—like a good life. Unlike denial, a healthy and secure base *scales*. As a society, if we develop a confident *inner* safety net as a public good, then it reflects for us all in a smart, risk-enabled populace with the willingness and ability to create in a free global economy. The increase is in our collective GNP and everyone's bottom line.

IF YOU ARE STILL BREATHING GAMBLE ON THAT WHICH WILL PROPEL you forward.

WHAT IF STEVE JOBS, AS AN ABANDONED CHILD, DID NOT FEEL worthy to risk and create Apple? Early on in his career, when he quit college, he might have *stayed* with calligraphy rather than the idea of making a world-dominating software and hardware design company. The ripples of monetary loss would be in the trillions of dollars in lost revenue. The ability to take risks is bone deep. Human development research and attachment theory says that: all of life is a series of daring adventures from a secure base. This framework, multiplied in time, incrementally governs an innovating (or stagnating) economy with diversifying skills, global connections and the basic risk-tolerant audacity to thrive in an uncertain world.

Right now, some new opportunity is growing in the dark—in the good dirt of our lives. Perhaps, it has been waiting for us to notice and nurture it for *a long time.*

An inherent belief in the goodness of the unseen is a bet worth placing.

28

BE CURIOUS

EVERY DAY CURIOSITY ALLOWS ME TO ACCURATELY BITE OFF WHAT I CAN CHEW.

We all place bets that will play out over time. How many wonderful things have happened to you in your life that you didn't plan? We pretend we have control over outcome but we do not.

OUR HUMAN INSTRUMENT PANEL LEVERAGES OUR ATTITUDES AND not much else. This is no small thing. It is a fulcrum that moves worlds.

Be Curious

MY MEMORY FILTER IS FOGGY. I HAVE FORGOTTEN MUCH OF THE minute-by-minute, drip, drip, drip decade of caregiving's uncertainties and stress.

I DO RECALL WITH CLARITY WAKING UP AT CERTAIN TIMES WHILE caring for my mother—frozen in overwhelm. Like a repeating dream of silent moments, I was the surfer *again* captured and stilled in a photo…as a whole ocean curled *around* me in a wave. I knew what was about to happen, and lacked any typically goofy-conquistador-like expression for the considerable skill of getting there (but twenty-four/seven caregiving is admittedly *master surfing…*). I knew I was about to explosively *become one* with a vast, crashing sea (and it was going to *hurt*).

HOW CAN I BE CURIOUS IF I SEE ONLY DISASTER (AND PERHAPS EVEN death) ahead?

IN CAREGIVING, MY FOCUS HAD NARROWED TO SUCH A DEGREE THAT any curiosity about what the day might bring had completely shut down. (I was a draft horse in blinders…) I had so little interest in what was not right in front of me that didn't even want to open the mail, much less answer the telephone. My coping skills at the time were a short list composed of avoidance and denial.

I NOTED IT ALL AND SIMPLY STASHED IT FOR PROCESSING…LATER. That later is now.

IT'S OKAY THAT IT TOOK SO LONG. IT SEEMS EVERY FEELING HAS A gestation-incubation period.

> "Everyone takes their time to be born and to die."
>
> — ANNA SENA DEFFENBAUGH STOWELL, MY GRANDMOTHER.

I have now learned to respect timing—more and more each day. There is a rightness—an order—about dealing with what shows up in my psychic in-box.

It's quantum housekeeping—noticing, receiving *curiously*, and sweeping it up. I am happy here, and ready for more. It is simply genius—to be curious.

> "I am neither clever nor particularly gifted, I am only very, very curious."
>
> —ALBERT EINSTEIN

Grief unraveled me—it can do the same for you. The trick is to allow it to do the heavy lifting.

Action may feel powerful. Not doing might feel wimpy and vulnerable but we need both. Sitting still is hard work for doers but easier when we ask ourselves how many wonderful things have happened to us, *not of our own doing?* (It's a long and joyfully unplanned list.) Eventually, I found a new normal, but I had to pass through an accumulation of unprocessed feelings. Not all of them. There are gifts here and unseen helpers. Grace happened but it is still messy work. We only have to take it in the bites, which we can manage. That's why it *Takes as Long as it Takes.* It's a *Joyous Wager* on a friendly Universe.

Do what you can, each day. Take a chewable bite of sadness, *if it is there for you.* Then take a walk, or do something on your happy list to recharge. *Stop. Rest,* if need be. Repeat as you can. Be gentle with yourself.

IT TOOK ME TIME TO BE CURIOUS AGAIN. CONSTRICTIONS AND FEAR are now a warning sign for me to pay attention...and be curious about what is going on *within* me.

BETTY MANAGED TO DRESS IN ST. JOHN'S KNITS ALL HER LIFE AND put food on the table, even if other people cooked it. For many of us who have been on the planet a while and have been gifted with *enough,* survival has *moved* to an inner arena. It's a great blessing to see this. I have enough food (I'm on a diet...); no one is shooting at me (and I *live* in Oakland...); I have a roof over my head (and a rose garden for smelling...); and many other mercies, which support me. My job now is to end suffering—in myself. Seeing with the *Gratitude of Redwoods* is working for me.

EVERY DAY CURIOSITY ALLOWS ME TO ACCURATELY BITE OFF WHAT I can chew.

MY OWN PURSUIT OF HAPPINESS IS TO GROW AN *INNER* ATTENTIVE lover, mother and father, which eases fear out of my driver's seat —*enough* for me to accept 'what is,' Enough for me to be curious again. I want life to be a dance with others—not a cross-country solo drive to get somewhere fast.

IT'S A LOT—TO FIND CURIOSITY AGAIN. IT'S EVERYTHING TO A GOOD life lived in an uncertain world.

29

UNLEARN CERTAINTY

CERTAINTY SELLS BUT IT DOESN'T ENDURE.

I have been longing for better stories—but haven't been able to tell them until now. I haven't been able to caregive better stories until now.

What Would Betty Say?

Healthy closure is an uneven thing—the only real criteria is that we, the bereaved, find a way to adjust our relationship with our lost one, in a way that gives us opportunity to live and love again. What that looks like is as unique as each of us.

Me, I have conversations with Betty—in absentia. I continued one of them, to catch her up on the time she had been gone from my sight. I was no longer a struggling, bootstrapped, cartographic Internet company founder. I am usually the last rat on the ship, but I quit. It was more than time.

I tried to sound nonchalant. "Oh, by the way I went to

seminary to become an Interfaith chaplain. I finished a residency at a hospital where I sat with the sick and dying, and their families. I've sat with Hindus, Buddhists, Hmong, evangelical and non-denominational Christians, Cabalists, Catholics, Jews, Native Americans, and more than a few Protestants. I have prayed with many of them. I have learned to support them in the tender human valleys that we will all be in at one time or another."

I TOOK A BREATH.

"I WAS THE ON-CALL CHAPLAIN WHO SHOWED UP AT SIX IN THE morning to the hospital room after a beautiful couple labored all night to deliver their stillborn baby. We blessed the baby—together. A week later I created and delivered a memorial service for that beautiful little unlit candle..."

I TOOK ANOTHER BREATH.

"ONE PARENT WAS FROM A HINDU FAMILY, THE OTHER FROM A Christian Orthodox one. They couldn't find a priest from either faith to honor *both* their traditions. I was privileged to be their last resort. I think it was the most wonderful thing I have ever done, second only to getting you to your end."

I TOOK ANOTHER BREATH...

"...AND I MARRIED MY SPIRITUAL-NOT-RELIGIOUS GODDAUGHTER and her agnostic groom on a beach in Carmel. I used quotes from

Einstein on love to leverage the secular into the sacred." I closed my eyes and saw my mother assessing me.

I CONTINUED, SAVING THE MOST SHOCKING FOR THE LAST, "...AND I have a job now as a full-time chaplain—*in hospice.* I am an *interfaith* chaplain. I support people of any faith or no faith and all the rivers that run between them."

THERE WAS SILENCE FOR A TIME, THEN SHE REPLIED, IMPENETRABLY, "I missed a lot in the last couple of years."

I CRITICALLY CORRECTED HER, "MORE LIKE SIX," THEN CAUGHT myself and softened it with a smile.

WHEN I TELL ACTUAL, *LIVING* FRIENDS ABOUT MY QUANTUM PIVOT they say something like, "Yeah, I can see that." Pretty much all my old dear friends took it as unsurprising and inferred.

"YOU HAVE ALWAYS BEEN THAT," SAID ONE OLD BEAU, WHO HAD known me for a lifetime and a half. More distant family friends say things like, "Betty would be so proud of you."

I'M NOT SO SURE. A MINISTERIAL DEGREE AND ORDINATION ONCE issued reduces your earning power by a third or more compared to any equivalent degree. I hear Betty's practical concerns mirroring her reactions to my first desires to be a painter.

'Good Enough' Dreams

By the omission of *my* time traveling vehicle of "when the business takes off," or "when my ship comes in" I have lost hope in the future and it is a good thing. The way I constantly lived in the future was saying here and now was not enough. I am less steering than doing a *Wait Here*—allowing the road to show itself. I began facing uncertainty—not avoiding the aspects of 'what is' that I wished would go away.

My mother did her avoidance by living in the past for much of our caregiving years by 'time-traveling' back to *anywhere else but where she was—sick and old.* During her illness, we met in paradoxical present tense moments—me living in the future and she in the past. *We waited it out, together—and got to here.*

I am here to become (or just remember) who I came here to be.

"Where do you see yourself in three years?" That's what I remember a perky twenty-something recruiter asked in a telephone screening soon after my mother died (and I was trying to figure out which way was up). It had been so long since I asked myself even that little question. Whatever I said was, apparently, too lame for a second telephone screening for the Google mapping job. (It wasn't mine to do...) I probably sounded lost because, of course, I was. I have found new worlds since then by allowing myself not to know. Not knowing is a *good thing* because what I used to know—for sure—is no longer true. All *my landmarks have changed*—there is no motherland to which (or to whom) I can run, kvetch, or cuddle. The business is done; I am stripped of any future hopes of a Secretariat-like-coming-from-behind kind of catch-up victory. I am a jockey without a horse. I do have goals, of course. I am my mother's daughter but they are more intention, at this point, than any real direction.

"WHAT ARE YOU DOING BUT USING OTHER PEOPLE'S NEEDS AS A substitute for having a compelling direction—the ex, mother, customers, cat…" My critic whispered this; there was no need to yell; it was beyond denial.

"ALL I WANTED FOR ELEVEN YEARS WAS TO HELP MY MOTHER OR TO serve my customers," I managed in my delivery of that statement, to not sound defensive. *I liked that*. "I did that well, damn it; those were massive accomplishments. I was fighting the good fight. I was in the arena. (I was Teddy Roosevelt's citizen in the republic…stumbling…but doing deeds…in the dust, the sweat and the blood... valiantly...striving…to a worthy cause…daring greatly…). Blah. Blah. Blah.

WHY DO I NOT FEEL MORE SATISFACTION?

"SO, WHAT DO I WANT?" I MUMBLED TO MYSELF WHO WAS (honestly) only half listening. "I want to pay off my credit cards which I racked up caregiving my mother, my business, and my cat."

BUT GETTING BACK TO ZERO, HARDLY SEEMS LIKE ENOUGH.

"OKAY, I WANT TO SAVE SOME MONEY SO I AM NOT SO STRESSED ALL the time and can be a better sister, auntie, and godmother."

STILL, THIS DID NOT SEEM LIKE ENOUGH.

"OKAY, I WANT TO BUY A HOUSE AND GO TO ITALY."

WELL, THAT WAS RIGHT OUT OF A GLOSSY GLAMOUR MAGAZINE. I should have big dreams but I am so beat up, I don't even remember my small ones.

"SO, WHAT DO I WANT?" IT IS THE MOST FUNDAMENTAL OF questions that you start asking at two years old. (At least I did.) In the terrible twos, I wanted candy. At four, I was more discerning and wanted pink candy. Then, as I got older, I wanted a pink room and pink clothes. Now, I can't stand pink.

WHAT I SEE IS THAT RIGHT WHERE I AM IS A PRETTY GREAT PLACE TO be. It's good enough. Right now is good enough. My life is quite amazing in its dailyness. It is a miraculous and mysterious alchemy of extraordinary ordinariness. My old world was about struggle and control but my new world is about resonance and finding a fit.

Unlearn Certainty

UNCERTAINTY EXPANDED WITH SO MANY DEATHS.

All my structures eroded: reliance on family, on a husband, on the efficacy of hard work's ability to move mountains. Death, divorce and unanticipated changed just happened. When so little of import, if anything, can be controlled or is truly *certain,* my ability to be *good* in the world evaporated. I wanted certainty, but it failed me.

CERTAINTY IS PERFECT KNOWLEDGE.
Certainty is freedom from error.
Certainty is fantasy.

CERTAINTY SELLS BUT IT DOESN'T ENDURE.

SURE, FOR A FEW QUARTERS AND TOUCHDOWNS IN LIFE, YOU MIGHT hold onto quarterback notions of controlling the forces of existence or being safe from gnarly vicissitudes. The mysteries of life and death, however, tend to be bruising offensive tackles (who, when in your face, are *very* hard to ignore).

CONFIDENCE, IN CONTRAST TO CERTAINTY, GROWS SLOWLY FROM within.

IT IS MORE A STATE OF BEING THAN DOING. CONFIDENCE MOVES US to bigger things by being successful at the incremental opportunities (and disasters). At its core, it is about *being* enough. Some parents give children an acorn-sized head start in loving acceptance. A blessing from an essential someone works, too. Other people, as myself, are offered the clarifying practice of good-self mothering/parenting. Whatever path brings you to enoughness, it accesses for us a resilience like the oak tree—strong yet flexible. Confidence is heartwood—growing a little more in fulfillment each season with an inner knowing that I am enough.

I CAN'T STEER WITH CERTAINTY IN WHITEWATER BUT I *CAN* POSITION myself for an eddy traveling my way.

I LEARNED TO UNLEARN WHAT WAS GETTING IN MY WAY. (SHAME OF not being enough, comes to mind...) When uncertainty expanded —into my lap—it became clear that I had never really developed confidence of my own—faking it but not actually making it.

TRUST THAT YOU'LL KNOW THE *VOICE* IN YOUR HEAD, WHEN YOU hear it (...It's the kind one).

LETTING GO OF CERTAINTIES (AND EVEN TENDING THEM LIKE A garden) gives me space to move and listen to a higher voice—and find resources overlooked before. It is not so much confidence *in my abilities,* but in the substance of things hoped for. This view invites curiosity, which allows us to grow better possibilities by finding evidence of things not seen—which had been hidden by the stress. Being appreciative of *what is,* confident in providential-just-in-time resources, gives me the strength and flexibility to *Be Curious* about *what's next.*

30

FEED ME FEEDBACK

IT'S ABOUT BEING WILLING TO TRY AGAIN, TO GROW AND BE BETTER—FROM INFORMATION RECEIVED.

My mother named me after herself—Elizabeth. It's uncertain if she was expecting the artistic female child born to her. Who or what she was hoping for in a daughter might have been a friend, a dynasty, or her own version 2.0.

HER WAR TO PROVE HERSELF NEVER HAD AN ARMISTICE. SHE NEVER rethought the battle strategy. She didn't change, or grow up and into the free will of choosing a *better* story for her own talents (much less seeing mine as a resource). As her lifelong observer, I experienced damage in her wake, but also bravery. She made beautiful (holy) sparks and responded to the magic of *her* moment —moving with the opportunities of *her times as she understood them to be.* She decided what kind of different she wanted, and she voted for it with her actions, and her considerable will. That's a lot to be proud of; I am proud of her. For the most part, she did as Emerson suggested:

> "Trust thyself: every heart vibrates to that iron

> string. Accept the place the divine providence has found for you, the society of your contemporaries, the connection of events. Great *(wo)*men have always done so, and confided themselves childlike to the genius of their age, betraying their perception that the absolutely trustworthy was seated at their heart, working through their hands, predominating in all their being."
>
> — RALPH WALDO EMERSON FROM SELF RELIANCE

CAREGIVING MY LIFE

It is my task to trust myself (and hum in harmony). How do I confide myself *'childlike to the genius of my age'* and believe that the *'absolutely trustworthy is seated at my heart?'* My answer is "Yes" but the question is the one, with which we started this field guide.

> "The most important question a person can ask is, "Is the Universe a friendly place?
>
> — ALBERT EINSTEIN

It is mine to ask and answer—so is it yours. The woman I knew as Mother would never understand that I have found work that I love on death's edge—the very edge that she spent her last eleven years fearfully avoiding. Maybe that was the plan all along —for me to find my own edge.

IF YOU ARE SUPPORTING A PERSON WHO IS ILL, OR ON DEMENTIA'S

death row, caregiving is not business as usual; it changes everything. It changes how we see time.

CAREGIVING IS *DANGEROUS* WORK. TO SURVIVE IT WELL, WE ARE asked to learn how to take care in operable ways that benefit everyone in attendance.

MY MOTHER AND I BEGAN AS FRACTURED AND GOT STUCK IN fractal—entangled in each other (even after her death). I tried to tend more than just her physical needs and to accompany her into time. The extended goodbye moved me out of the Newtonian and into the unknown because tending a dying loved one places you in the nether world of grief, *years before they die.* We lose them in such small increments and their dying takes so long, it is easy to bury or misplace vast pieces of you, too (but perhaps that, too, is part of it). The quantum enveloped us and only my long, rotten road of grief healed me. *It benefitted me*. Parts of me stayed lost.

THE PARTS THAT ARE MINE I WILL CONTINUE TO RECLAIM. OTHER pieces are buried with her, and will pass from my life (with continued *Right Weeding).*

IT MAKES SENSE. MY BODY BEGAN AS A SINGLE CELL WITHIN HERS, dividing and separating its way out. After a lifetime of transformation, it proved not enough and her life fell into *my* care. Death itself was not enough to separate us—not really. We are now complete. It is enough. She is now safely *within me.*

SHE IS HOME AND I AM TOO. I AM HOME IN MY OWN LIFE AND SKIN, doing what is mine to do. Parts of what I thought were 'me' have passed away. The story that was *in me,* was *not* me. At this point, it feels like a mistaken identity...amnesia or...a cosmic joke, in which I somehow missed the punchline for years.

I AM RIGHT WHERE (AND WHEN) I AM MEANT TO BE.

Feed Me Feedback

HOW DO I STAY ATTUNED TO WHAT IS MINE TO DO?

Finding the information given to me from the cranky, and well-intentioned is not easy. The linkage that makes me renewable is being able to course correct. This is fertile soil but it must be regularly amended and even tilled.

BOTH RULES, *MAGIC METTLE* AND *GOT BLESSING?*, ARE THE quantum compost to do this. It allows us enough confidence to hear and receive data amid the annoying words of uncle whoever's criticism...*and dump the rest* into the good earth (which knows what to do with it). This regenerates us in the (booms and) busts of the trenches. It grows resiliency and allows us to bounce—and, perhaps, get to a flirtatious, happy hundredth year—like a resilient Olga and Madeline, a feisty Albertina and Alpha or a beatific and forgiving Alice.

WE ARE NOT MADE TO DO THIS ALONE.

We need our fellow passengers, our time-traveling shipmates, to help us refine the implementations of our dreams. We don't do great ventures by ourselves—contrary to the prairie rugged individualist grit (...useful in sprints, but not a marathon). When my manifest-destiny burdened ancestors finally got to the Pacific after cheating, killing, stealing (and working their butts off) all the way West, we hit the coast and had no more landscapes to conquer but ourselves. One life at a time, we have been trying to figure ourselves out ever since—taking feedback is the key. *It is the basis of all innovation*—and what makes the Golden State *gold* (and the Pacific Northwest green) because we don't do great things alone. We need each other.

It's ABOUT BEING WILLING TO TRY AGAIN, TO GROW AND BE BETTER —from information received.

JUST BECAUSE I *LISTEN* TO ADVICE DOESN'T MEAN I TAKE IT, BUT IT could be the key to discovering something *wonderful*. Feedback is easier to accept if it is tactful—but even if unskillful, if it lands on the fertile, adult soil of willingness (not narcissistic willfulness) it can be course correcting. *You can pivot.* Changing how a dream looks (or starting again from scratch) may be the quickest and best way to get to where you want to be. It is the difference between persistence and stubbornness (which can be look-a-likes). I lost a lot not receiving feedback well.

RECOGNIZING THAT WE DON'T KNOW IT ALL, AND *BEING WILLING* TO see another's viewpoint, or even how you see me (or it) allows us to craft a better story that fits the way *it is now*.

BETTER QUESTIONS RULE IN CREATIVE VENTURES AND THE GOOD life. What fits?

WHAT DO YOU WANT—NOW? PLANT IT. ADD A BLESSING AND (*Mangia, Mangia)* eat the good word-food that pleases *your* palette, ground it with *Feed Me Feedback.*

LISTEN TO THE NEW LIFE SPEAKING TO YOU IN YOUR OWN VOICE.

NO SHUSSING. REMEMBER...BETTER.

31

ONE STORY

HUMAN BEINGS ARE POWERED BY STORIES...A LOVE STORY.

What I know for sure about Betty's husbands is simple. There were five of them and she married for love. She was in love, then, a year (or years) later, was *not*. It's our human story. It seems that once we get on the planet, we begin exploring the road that love is and the potholes of what it is not. Usually, we must leave home to do it. Perhaps there are humans who can stay put and explore. The lovely blue bird of happiness sings for them *where they are*...and they don't feel *enough* discontent or restlessness to move.

THESE PEOPLE DO *NOT* BELONG TO MY FAMILY.

I SEE CHOICES IN ANY GIVEN MOMENT AS A CONTINUUM OF LOVE TO fear. I have inherited fear-based ideas and have personally honed others. Fear has shown up in my life and taken over, but fear will always be there. The right question in any given moment is can I choose more love? How do I choose more love from the feast on my banquet table? It may be the only question my life needs to answer—ever. More love? Or less love? More kindness or… less?

HOW CAN I EXPAND THE CAPACITY OF MY HEART TO ACCEPT, understand, and have compassion for myself and others?

> "There is no fear where love exists. Rather, perfect love banishes fear, for fear involves punishment, and the person who lives in fear has not been perfected in love."
>
> — 1 JOHN 4:18 ISV

No fear in caregiving (or any other edgy human endeavor) would be nice—but tactically unlikely. Courage is doing what we do, in spite of the fear. Every superhero (or caregiver) knows this. However, in the trenches the more love I have the less fear, I can hold. Thich Nhat Hanh likens the human heart to an immense river. If we have enough flow of love, little bothers us and little pollutes us. He speaks the most important question, how do we help our hearts to grow in capacity (and flow) like a river?

HOW DO WE HOLD MORE LOVE AND STOP THE LEAKS? I HAVE noticed my own leaks—that comfort for dwelling in the dramatic nuances of my righteous wounding or resentments where I blame others for outcomes. (The ones where I am right and *they* are wrong.) Yet, when I have enough, I can overlook anything. It's an inner balance. Remember when you were "in love", did it matter where they left their dirty socks? Or any other nit picky thing?

IT'S OUR HUMAN STORY. LONG OR SHORT, EVERY HUMAN LIFETIME seems to be just one story. It's a love story.

CAREGIVING EPIPHANIES

There is a moment in every long goodbye when a caregiver 'gets' it. There is no going back; we know it will never be 'normal' again. There is no more denial or even hoping: your loved one is more gone than with you.

FOR THE FIVE YEARS WE LIVED TOGETHER, I ACTED AND REACTED, AS if Betty would heal. It took me a long time to realize that she would not. We had dinner parties in which she happily presided at the head of the table *but was unusually silent.* We went through a lot of egg poacher pans, which she forgot on the gas stove until the smoke sensors alerted us. It got worse as we lived together, not better. Things settled down after the couple of years of catastrophic illnesses, frequent ER visits, and her early grief over the death of my brother. Diminished, she became a CPA who could no longer balance her own checkbook. My brother's death made her not care.

"I GOT A NEW CLIENT TODAY, WILL YOU HELP ME DO HIS TAXES?"

IT WAS MATH HOMEWORK HELL ALL OVER AGAIN BUT WITH NO *RIGHT* answers. I helped her, too, because at that point I still thought she would get through it and be the Betty I used to know. I see this at bedside as a hospice chaplain—my own time of utter cluelessness reflected back at me. My experience inside the magical-thinking bubble—fearfully hoping beyond all evidence that *this* change was not happening—gifts me with endless empathy for the loving vacillations of families on this edge. It takes time to *know it's time.*

GRAVITY CHANGED

I continued to get angry with her when I thought she was not trying hard enough to improve...until the day when gravity completely shifted. It was a bad day—probably like the bad day the dinosaurs had when their end-of-life comet hit the Earth. It was four years into my caregiving, with seven more to go.

"HONEY, YOU NEED TO TAKE BETTER CARE OF YOURSELF." I, THE POT, instructed the kettle. She, the cosmetic queen, had not cleansed her face in a long while and more shockingly had not put on any night cream.

"HOW ABOUT YOU BRUSH YOUR TEETH AND PUT SOME OF THAT lovely cream on your face. If feels quite dry." I ran my hand over her cheek very gently and smiled at her. She said she would. I remember that moment as very tender. There was no resistance in her...the oddity of that did not register until later.

THE NEXT MORNING, SHE CAME OUT OF HER ROOM ALL DRESSED FOR her *New York Times* morning ritual as was her habit in our daily-ness. Her place was in her rocker, by the corner window, over-looking the Presidio and the Pacific. As she walked toward me, I prepared to execute a pre-emptive strike on her daily-poached eggs on toast, offering to make them for her and save the new pan from fresh torture. I paused. On her face, I saw some white cream, which had not been completely absorbed.

I SAID TO HER, "OH, GOOD FOR YOU, MY DARLING, YOU PUT SOME cream on your..."

I TOUCHED HER CHEEK TO FINISH RUBBING IN THE CREAM. IT WAS hard and crusty. Then I smelled...spearmint. It was *toothpaste.*

I STARTED TEARING UP. I HUGGED HER SO SHE COULDN'T SEE. *MY* mother—the madam of makeup—could not tell the difference between face cream and toothpaste...or the *smell* or the *feel* of it drying on her face. Up to that moment, I could not conceive of a world where that *might be.* No parallel universe could *possibly* exist to be that weird. Paint was dripping sideways and gravity was no longer a constant.

LIKE THE DINOSAURS, I NEVER SAW IT COMING.

MY FIGHT TO *FIX* HER STOPPED *IN THAT MOMENT*—THE QUANTUM Toothpaste Pivot. I ceased fighting. There was no one to fight with—no worthy opposition. In place of the struggle, compassion flooded in. I don't know how all the anger died and I don't know from where all the kindness arrived but from that second everything changed. I began a very different relationship with my mother as the only adult in the room.

FROM THIS VANTAGE POINT, I SEE EVERY HUMAN KNUCKLEHEAD AS doing the best he/she/we can. Having said that, this rule is a handy metric that has guided me closer to a place of balance between the broken extremes of denial and excess. This is particularly important when caregiving.

One Story

HUMAN BEINGS ARE POWERED BY STORIES...A LOVE STORY

We need them to live. When a loved one dies, a story ends. As I was, we can be mistaken about what stories are ours and which ones belong to someone else. Whether the story was still good for me or not, it remains a shock to have it taken *from you* by an illness or a death or some other change not of my making. We can make new stories or end the ones that no longer serve us. Seeing life as a series of love stories or really just one human story, I can more easily listen to my God-given longings and discontents. They are mysterious plot lines and guides to what my next chapter might be. Opportunities to choose a better story start here.

OUR STORIES ARE *NOT* THE BOSSES OF US (AND NEITHER IS OUR DNA for that matter). All major religions and all the spiritual mystics say that love is the boss of us. I want to side with love—the most I can muster in any given moment and make love live *in my story.*

BETTY CHOSE LOVE—AS SHE HOPED IT WOULD BE—FROM HER experience. *She chose—but love isn't* black and white. Love isn't a hopeful, greeting card sentiment; it is a superpower of holding opposites. Love changes color and shape over time. (She loved me and did a not-too-good a job of showing me, early on.)

IN THE TOUGH AND TENDER TRENCHES, THE MORE LOVING CHOICE might only have a twinkle of difference (or holy spark, if you're paying attention) between more love or more fear.

HOW DO WE KEEP SIDING WITH MORE LOVE (AND NOT FEAR) IN OUR next moment?

IMBEDDED AND UNDERGIRDING BETTER DECISIONS ARE THE *MAGIC Mettle* of confidence in providence...and in oneself. It is the way to better navigation in the paradoxical caregiver's world between 'shit happens' and assurances that 'it will *all* be okay.' Then we can accept the challenges of the day: war, battle, strife, loss, disappointments, depressions, wacky parenting, knuckle headed loving, and bad hair days. After all nuance, avoidance, vacillation, bifurcation and distraction, we have this choice: align with love or fear. It's simple, but not easy.

> "'Love the Lord your God with all your heart and with all your soul and with all your mind.' This is the first and greatest commandment. And the second is like it: 'Love your neighbor as yourself.' All the Law and the Prophets hang on these two commandments."
>
> — MATTHEW 22: 37 NIV

In the past, I have needed (and made-up) enemies (jumping over the Biblical fine print of loving them) by refusing to see that we are all doing *the best we can here*. We are all choosing the better over the worse—*as we understand it to be.*

EVEN IF IT DOESN'T *LOOK* LIKE A LOVE STORY, I SEE LOVE AS THE *author* of this play.

Check into *your caregiving* moment with good *caring* questions.

Is fear more dominant now? Or does this choice make more love in my world? Am I doing the right thing for the wrong reason? Did I care for Betty because it was honorable? Did I want something from her that I hadn't yet gotten? Or both? Or, here's a personal favorite, am I stuck in the narcissism of a child, scared that I will not have enough toys and other good stuff for myself? Or the ultimate caregiver question, what would *they* want? It's easy to pull my own fear and pain avoidance strategies into the story. My mother was ready to leave this world long before I was willing to let her go.

Statistically, this is common. We caregivers want our beloveds to fight when they would rather rest because we, ourselves, are scared. To be fair, few of our seriously ill elders make their preferences known on paper (...that would be an Advanced Directive). A good end is truthful. What does your loved one want for a good end? The question is clarifying. It gives you the gift of knowing—not guessing. This is one of the most fertile of soils upon which we, their caregivers, can plant an honorable future.

Caregiving with love and good questions changes the planet.

What does love want? What do you want for your love story? I have seen love change shape in the moment and completely flip the plot around. 'Villains' become heroes; heroes show their humanity and the ordinary becomes an extraordinary gemstone. I see love showing us the way—and it always has.

LIVE YOUR LOVE STORY...LIKE YOUR OWN GOOD LIFE DEPENDS upon it.

~

Knowing you are enough,
May you feel the good food in your veins,
May you use all the gifts that you have been given...to widen your circle of care.

We need you here...the world wants you here.

Thank you for all you do.

~

EPILOG

Reading caregiving memoirs while you are actively caregiving or freshly grieving may be tender. It may feel better to tell and retell *your own story* for a time—to get your bearings and *to make it real.* I recommend a good grief group, a bereavement counselor, or good friends who know the value of listening. Actually, all of the above is even better. Contact your hospice provider (or any hospice provider) for grief counseling or groups. It is their job (and privilege) to support you.

If this is where you find yourself, I invite you to sign up for our bereavement newsletter.

The Garden of Change Bereavement Newsletter has been designed to support people who need actionable information in a body-mind-spirit approach with, perhaps, a bit of spiritual perspective on grief. An Interfaith perspective balanced with what current research (and the ancient wise) know about getting through grief in a healthy way. Many hospices use it to support their families.

If you are a hospice, we can help you, too at www.gardenofchange.org.

Thank you and blessings on your journey.

Rev. EM

THE MEMOIR

GIRLQUANTUM—A TIME-TRAVELING MEMOIR OF A BETTER REMEMBERING

The Memoir: *girlQuantum*

When we are in our own tender valleys of caregiving, we may or may not find other people's stories about *their* comparative caregiving challenges all that helpful. In fact, it can be very painful and confusing. Have you experienced an acquaintance or a friend ask you how you are, and as you open your mouth to say, they launch into *their own* story of a similar experience? They are themselves still grieving and may not even know it.

AFTER YOU HAVE ACCOMPLISHED YOUR GOALS AND GOTTEN caregiving behind you, (either your sweet old someone is now well, or has safely moved on and into the great mystery), you will be okay. (Their outcome is not up to you, only the love that you have shared is on your plate.) However, if you are ready and curious to know how the gifts in the field guide came about, I invite you into our larger story. The story is context for my rules. Our story time-travels because my mother did. It was also a prize-fight. Our lifelong argument erupted as many things, but at its core, there was only one—a worldview: Betty's vs. mine. It was intimate and public: confused and loud. It was a multi-year, many-round championship boxing match, which we had from Tulsa to San Francisco, over the answer to this question:

> "The most important question a person can ask is, "Is the Universe a friendly place?"
>
> — ALBERT EINSTEIN

I say yes. The rules help me remember that friendly providence in the garden of change.

GIRLQUANTUM—THE TIME-TRAVELING MEMOIR OF A BETTER Remembering (...the *next* book)

If you wish to know more of the story of my mother and me, which generated *A Hospice Chaplain's Field Guide to Caregiving,* I invite you into the book of our journey. As is every caregiving journey, and it is completely unique and common to all of us. I invite you to join us for a digital and serial rollout. You will find out more at www.EMHager.com.

APPENDIX

THE 31 GIFTS—A SUMMARY

Gift No.1 Wait Here Stop struggling. Wait Here for the goodness to catch up.

Gift No. 2 Stay Full *Running on empty? Stay full to do what is yours to do today...that's enough.*

Gift No. 3 Etak Compass *Our longings and discontents are inner guidance.*

Gift No. 4 Diva Breathe Generous people breathe deep but real divas let it go. Think Pavarotti.

Gift No. 5. The Gratitude of Redwoods Allow gratitude to turn what you have into enough.

Gift No. 6 Play Daily Playing right where I am is the long game—especially in the leftover moments.

Gift No. 7 Be Willing *If I am willing, I am not broken.*

Gift No. 8 Stop. Rest Take off your cape. Decisions will be made—but not right now.

Gift No. 9 Flash Light Name the fear. It's a light switch—light on and fear off.

Gift No.10 Bounce Well *Bounce is an ethos...and cyclical.*

Gift No. 11 Mangia, Mangia Fast food or slow food, choose to make it real food to fuel your life.

Gift No. 12 Bedrock Allowing *Allow the 'imperfect' in. It may, given a chance, appreciate you back.*

Gift No.13 Lean Back *Lean back into waiting arms—see who is still there when you do.*

Gift No. 14 It Takes as Long as it Takes Grit is insanely useful in caregiving, but in grief—not so much.

Gift No.15. Keep Moving *Allow providence to flow to you and through you. Take the next step, even if small.*

Gift No.16 Do Bother *Woven under the surface of things, love wants to be bothered with your troubles.*

Gift No.17. Cackle *Call up the "Evil" Queen (in your grievance story du jour). Say you're buying dinner.*

Gift No.18. Phoenix Carousel Inspire a renewal—light the match. Even if you think it's your last one.

Gift No.19 Celebrate Inconvenience Double-down with fun in the middle of the messiness.

Gift No. 20 Live Backwards, Remember Better *Memory is a garden. What and how I choose to remember grows my life.*

Gift No. 21 Mobius Regrets *Congratulate yourself. Regrets can be an infinite loop to better.*

Gift No. 22 Improv "What is" *Underneath all the chaos of "What is", love waits to play.*

Gift No. 23 Magic Mettle *Try these magic words: "What you are is already awesome.' Welcome home.*

Gift No. 24 Got Blessing? Validation is for parking—but having a blessing is a constantly refilling gas tank.

Gift No. 25 Wild Within *Now is the time for wildness, temperance....and laughter—dreaming a little wilder and wider.*

Gift No. 26 Right Weeding *What's the difference between a weed and a flower? It's a lot like real estate.*

Gift No. 27 Joyous Wager *An inherent belief in the goodness of the unseen is a bet worth placing.*

Gift No. 28. Be Curious *Every day curiosity allows me to accurately bite off what I can chew.*

Gift No.29 Unlearn Certainty *Certainty sells but it doesn't endure.*

Gift No. 30 Feed Me Feedback *It's* about being willing to try again, to grow and be better—from information received.

Gift No. 31 One Story *Human beings are powered by stories...a love story.*

END NOTES

Gift 4—Diva Breathe

Endnote 1—From *"Breathing as if Your Life Depended Upon It,"* by *Psychology Today* Blog Writer Steve Sisgold, June 12, 2012 https://www.psychologytoday.com/blog/life-in-body/201206/breathe-your-life-depends-it

Gift 5—The Gratitude of Redwoods

Endnote 2—From *"The Upward Spiral* Using Neuroscience to Reverse the Course of Depression, One Small Change at Time," by Alex Korb, PhD. Copyright 2015, published by New Harbinger Publications, Inc.

Endnote 3—From Professor Suzanne Simard talks about *"Mother Trees"* Excerpt from University of British Columbia Reports UBC Reports, Vol 57, No. 7, 2011. http://www.forestry.ubc.ca/2011/05/prof-suzanne-simard-talks-about-mother-trees/

Gift 6—Play Daily

End Note 4– www.MakingSpaceSacred.com

Gift 22—Improv "What is"

End Note 5 —From *"In Service of Life"* by Rachel Naomi Remen, *Noetic Sciences Review* # 37 Spring 1996

End Note 6 —From *"This American Life"* Act Two, Rainey Days and Mondys

https://www.thisamericanlife.org/radio-archives/episode/532/magic-words Producer Chana Joffe-Walt interviews Karen Stobbe and her husband Mondy about a plan they've recently enacted in their family. Karen's mother lives with them and she has dementia. Karen and Mondy are actors and they stumbled upon a skill they have that is incredibly useful in communicating with Karen's mother – improv. http://www.in-themoment.com/

Gift 23 Magic Mettle

End Note 7 —Unconditional positive regard, a concept developed by the humanistic psychologist Carl Rogers, is the basic acceptance and support of a person regardless of what the person says or does.

Gift 26 Right Weeding

End Note 8 – From Matthew 13:3-9

33681169R00113

Made in the USA
Middletown, DE
17 January 2019